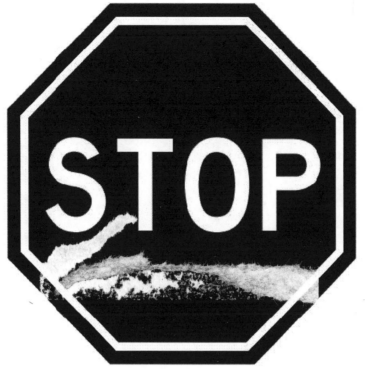

FREE Test Taking Tips DVD Offer

To help us better serve you, we have developed a Test Taking Tips DVD that we would like to give you for FREE. **This DVD covers world-class test taking tips that you can use to be even more successful when you are taking your test.**

All that we ask is that you email us your feedback about your study guide. Please let us know what you thought about it – whether that is good, bad or indifferent.

To get your **FREE Test Taking Tips DVD**, email freedvd@studyguideteam.com with "FREE DVD" in the subject line and the following information in the body of the email:

    a. The title of your study guide.

    b. Your product rating on a scale of 1-5, with 5 being the highest rating.

    c. Your feedback about the study guide. What did you think of it?

    d. Your full name and shipping address to send your free DVD.

If you have any questions or concerns, please don't hesitate to contact us at freedvd@studyguideteam.com.

Thanks again!

HESI A2 Study Questions 2018 & 2019

Three Full-Length HESI A2 Practice Tests: 900+ Test Prep Questions for the HESI Admission Assessment 4th Edition Exam

HESI A2 Study Guide 2018 & 2019 Prep Team

Table of Contents

Quick Overview

As you draw closer to taking your exam, effective preparation becomes more and more important. Thankfully, you have this study guide to help you get ready. Use this guide to help keep your studying on track and refer to it often.

This study guide contains several key sections that will help you be successful on your exam. The guide contains tips for what you should do the night before and the day of the test. Also included are test-taking tips. Knowing the right information is not always enough. Many well-prepared test takers struggle with exams. These tips will help equip you to accurately read, assess, and answer test questions.

A large part of the guide is devoted to showing you what content to expect on the exam and to helping you better understand that content. Near the end of this guide is a practice test so that you can see how well you have grasped the content. Then, answer explanations are provided so that you can understand why you missed certain questions.

Don't try to cram the night before you take your exam. This is not a wise strategy for a few reasons. First, your retention of the information will be low. Your time would be better used by reviewing information you already know rather than trying to learn a lot of new information. Second, you will likely become stressed as you try to gain a large amount of knowledge in a short amount of time. Third, you will be depriving yourself of sleep. So be sure to go to bed at a reasonable time the night before. Being well-rested helps you focus and remain calm.

Be sure to eat a substantial breakfast the morning of the exam. If you are taking the exam in the afternoon, be sure to have a good lunch as well. Being hungry is distracting and can make it difficult to focus. You have hopefully spent lots of time preparing for the exam. Don't let an empty stomach get in the way of success!

When travelling to the testing center, leave earlier than needed. That way, you have a buffer in case you experience any delays. This will help you remain calm and will keep you from missing your appointment time at the testing center.

Be sure to pace yourself during the exam. Don't try to rush through the exam. There is no need to risk performing poorly on the exam just so you can leave the testing center early. Allow yourself to use all of the allotted time if needed.

Remain positive while taking the exam even if you feel like you are performing poorly. Thinking about the content you should have mastered will not help you perform better on the exam.

Once the exam is complete, take some time to relax. Even if you feel that you need to take the exam again, you will be well served by some down time before you begin studying again. It's often easier to convince yourself to study if you know that it will come with a reward!

Test-Taking Strategies

1. Predicting the Answer

When you feel confident in your preparation for a multiple-choice test, try predicting the answer before reading the answer choices. This is especially useful on questions that test objective factual knowledge or that ask you to fill in a blank. By predicting the answer before reading the available choices, you eliminate the possibility that you will be distracted or led astray by an incorrect answer choice. You will feel more confident in your selection if you read the question, predict the answer, and then find your prediction among the answer choices. After using this strategy, be sure to still read all of the answer choices carefully and completely. If you feel unprepared, you should not attempt to predict the answers. This would be a waste of time and an opportunity for your mind to wander in the wrong direction.

2. Reading the Whole Question

Too often, test takers scan a multiple-choice question, recognize a few familiar words, and immediately jump to the answer choices. Test authors are aware of this common impatience, and they will sometimes prey upon it. For instance, a test author might subtly turn the question into a negative, or he or she might redirect the focus of the question right at the end. The only way to avoid falling into these traps is to read the entirety of the question carefully before reading the answer choices.

3. Looking for Wrong Answers

Long and complicated multiple-choice questions can be intimidating. One way to simplify a difficult multiple-choice question is to eliminate all of the answer choices that are clearly wrong. In most sets of answers, there will be at least one selection that can be dismissed right away. If the test is administered on paper, the test taker could draw a line through it to indicate that it may be ignored; otherwise, the test taker will have to perform this operation mentally or on scratch paper. In either case, once the obviously incorrect answers have been eliminated, the remaining choices may be considered. Sometimes identifying the clearly wrong answers will give the test taker some information about the correct answer. For instance, if one of the remaining answer choices is a direct opposite of one of the eliminated answer choices, it may well be the correct answer. The opposite of obviously wrong is obviously right! Of course, this is not always the case. Some answers are obviously incorrect simply because they are irrelevant to the question being asked. Still, identifying and eliminating some incorrect answer choices is a good way to simplify a multiple-choice question.

4. Don't Overanalyze

Anxious test takers often overanalyze questions. When you are nervous, your brain will often run wild, causing you to make associations and discover clues that don't actually exist. If you feel that this may be a problem for you, do whatever you can to slow down during the test. Try taking a deep breath or counting to ten. As you read and consider the question, restrict yourself to the particular words used by the author. Avoid thought tangents about what the author *really* meant, or what he or she was *trying* to say. The only things that matter on a multiple-choice test are the words that are actually in the question. You must avoid reading too much into a multiple-choice question, or supposing that the writer meant something other than what he or she wrote.

5. No Need for Panic

It is wise to learn as many strategies as possible before taking a multiple-choice test, but it is likely that you will come across a few questions for which you simply don't know the answer. In this situation, avoid panicking. Because most multiple-choice tests include dozens of questions, the relative value of a single wrong answer is small. Moreover, your failure on one question has no effect on your success elsewhere on the test. As much as possible, you should compartmentalize each question on a multiple-choice test. In other words, you should not allow your feelings about one question to affect your success on the others. When you find a question that you either don't understand or don't know how to answer, just take a deep breath and do your best. Read the entire question slowly and carefully. Try rephrasing the question a couple of different ways. Then, read all of the answer choices carefully. After eliminating obviously wrong answers, make a selection and move on to the next question.

6. Confusing Answer Choices

When working on a difficult multiple-choice question, there may be a tendency to focus on the answer choices that are the easiest to understand. Many people, whether consciously or not, gravitate to the answer choices that require the least concentration, knowledge, and memory. This is a mistake. When you come across an answer choice that is confusing, you should give it extra attention. A question might be confusing because you do not know the subject matter to which it refers. If this is the case, don't eliminate the answer before you have affirmatively settled on another. When you come across an answer choice of this type, set it aside as you look at the remaining choices. If you can confidently assert that one of the other choices is correct, you can leave the confusing answer aside. Otherwise, you will need to take a moment to try to better understand the confusing answer choice. Rephrasing is one way to tease out the sense of a confusing answer choice.

7. Your First Instinct

Many people struggle with multiple-choice tests because they overthink the questions. If you have studied sufficiently for the test, you should be prepared to trust your first instinct once you have carefully and completely read the question and all of the answer choices. There is a great deal of research suggesting that the mind can come to the correct conclusion very quickly once it has obtained all of the relevant information. At times, it may seem to you as if your intuition is working faster even than your reasoning mind. This may in fact be true. The knowledge you obtain while studying may be retrieved from your subconscious before you have a chance to work out the associations that support it. Verify your instinct by working out the reasons that it should be trusted.

8. Key Words

Many test takers struggle with multiple-choice questions because they have poor reading comprehension skills. Quickly reading and understanding a multiple-choice question requires a mixture of skill and experience. To help with this, try jotting down a few key words and phrases on a piece of scrap paper. Doing this concentrates the process of reading and forces the mind to weigh the relative importance of the question's parts. In selecting words and phrases to write down, the test taker thinks about the question more deeply and carefully. This is especially true for multiple-choice questions that are preceded by a long prompt.

9. Subtle Negatives

One of the oldest tricks in the multiple-choice test writer's book is to subtly reverse the meaning of a question with a word like *not* or *except*. If you are not paying attention to each word in the question, you can easily be led astray by this trick. For instance, a common question format is, "Which of the following is...?" Obviously, if the question instead is, "Which of the following is not...?," then the answer will be quite different. Even worse, the test makers are aware of the potential for this mistake and will include one answer choice that would be correct if the question were not negated or reversed. A test taker who misses the reversal will find what he or she believes to be a correct answer and will be so confident that he or she will fail to reread the question and discover the original error. The only way to avoid this is to practice a wide variety of multiple-choice questions and to pay close attention to each and every word.

10. Reading Every Answer Choice

It may seem obvious, but you should always read every one of the answer choices! Too many test takers fall into the habit of scanning the question and assuming that they understand the question because they recognize a few key words. From there, they pick the first answer choice that answers the question they believe they have read. Test takers who read all of the answer choices might discover that one of the latter answer choices is actually *more* correct. Moreover, reading all of the answer choices can remind you of facts related to the question that can help you arrive at the correct answer. Sometimes, a misstatement or incorrect detail in one of the latter answer choices will trigger your memory of the subject and will enable you to find the right answer. Failing to read all of the answer choices is like not reading all of the items on a restaurant menu: you might miss out on the perfect choice.

11. Spot the Hedges

One of the keys to success on multiple-choice tests is paying close attention to every word. This is never more true than with words like *almost*, *most*, *some*, and *sometimes*. These words are called "hedges" because they indicate that a statement is not totally true or not true in every place and time. An absolute statement will contain no hedges, but in many subjects, like literature and history, the answers are not always straightforward or absolute. There are always exceptions to the rules in these subjects. For this reason, you should favor those multiple-choice questions that contain hedging language. The presence of qualifying words indicates that the author is taking special care with his or her words, which is certainly important when composing the right answer. After all, there are many ways to be wrong, but there is only one way to be right! For this reason, it is wise to avoid answers that are absolute when taking a multiple-choice test. An absolute answer is one that says things are either all one way or all another. They often include words like *every*, *always*, *best*, and *never*. If you are taking a multiple-choice test in a subject that doesn't lend itself to absolute answers, be on your guard if you see any of these words.

12. Long Answers

In many subject areas, the answers are not simple. As already mentioned, the right answer often requires hedges. Another common feature of the answers to a complex or subjective question are qualifying clauses, which are groups of words that subtly modify the meaning of the sentence. If the question or answer choice describes a rule to which there are exceptions or the subject matter is complicated, ambiguous, or confusing, the correct answer will require many words in order to be expressed clearly and accurately. In essence, you should not be deterred by answer choices that seem excessively long. Oftentimes, the author of the text will not be able to write the correct answer without offering some qualifications and modifications. Your job is to read the answer choices thoroughly and completely and to select the one that most accurately and precisely answers the question.

13. Restating to Understand

Sometimes, a question on a multiple-choice test is difficult not because of what it asks but because of how it is written. If this is the case, restate the question or answer choice in different words. This process serves a couple of important purposes. First, it forces you to concentrate on the core of the question. In order to rephrase the question accurately, you have to understand it well. Rephrasing the question will concentrate your mind on the key words and ideas. Second, it will present the information to your mind in a fresh way. This process may trigger your memory and render some useful scrap of information picked up while studying.

14. True Statements

Sometimes an answer choice will be true in itself, but it does not answer the question. This is one of the main reasons why it is essential to read the question carefully and completely before proceeding to the answer choices. Too often, test takers skip ahead to the answer choices and look for true statements. Having found one of these, they are content to select it without reference to the question above. Obviously, this provides an easy way for test makers to play tricks. The savvy test taker will always read the entire question before turning to the answer choices. Then, having settled on a correct answer choice, he or she will refer to the original question and ensure that the selected answer is relevant. The mistake of choosing a correct-but-irrelevant answer choice is especially common on questions related to specific pieces of objective knowledge, like historical or scientific facts. A prepared test taker will have a wealth of factual knowledge at his or her disposal, and should not be careless in its application.

15. No Patterns

One of the more dangerous ideas that circulates about multiple-choice tests is that the correct answers tend to fall into patterns. These erroneous ideas range from a belief that B and C are the most common right answers, to the idea that an unprepared test-taker should answer "A-B-A-C-A-D-A-B-A." It cannot be emphasized enough that pattern-seeking of this type is exactly the WRONG way to approach a multiple-choice test. To begin with, it is highly unlikely that the test maker will plot the correct answers according to some predetermined pattern. The questions are scrambled and delivered in a random order. Furthermore, even if the test maker was following a pattern in the assignation of correct answers, there is no reason why the test taker would know which pattern he or she was using. Any attempt to discern a pattern in the answer choices is a waste of time and a distraction from the real work of taking the test. A test taker would be much better served by extra preparation before the test than by reliance on a pattern in the answers.

FREE DVD OFFER

Don't forget that doing well on your exam includes both understanding the test content and understanding how to use what you know to do well on the test. We offer a completely FREE Test Taking Tips DVD that covers world class test taking tips that you can use to be even more successful when you are taking your test.

All that we ask is that you email us your feedback about your study guide. To get your **FREE Test Taking Tips DVD**, email freedvd@studyguideteam.com with "FREE DVD" in the subject line and the following information in the body of the email:

- The title of your study guide.
- Your product rating on a scale of 1-5, with 5 being the highest rating.
- Your feedback about the study guide. What did you think of it?
- Your full name and shipping address to send your free DVD.

Introduction to the HESI Admission Assessment Exam

Function of the Test

The Health Education Systems, Inc. (HESI) Admission Assessment (A2) Exam is an entrance exam intended for high school graduates seeking admission to post-secondary health programs such as nursing schools. Test-takers have typically not received any training in specific medical subjects. The test is offered nationwide by the colleges and universities that require it as part of an applicant's admission package.

Test Administration

Many of the specifics of the process of HESI administration are determined at the discretion of the testing institution. For instance, each school may choose to administer the entire HESI exam or any portion thereof. Accordingly, there is no set process or schedule for taking the exam; instead, the schedule is determined on a case-by-case basis by the institution administering the exam. Likewise, the cost of the HESI is set by the administering institution. The typical cost is usually around $40-$70.

Find out ahead of time which sections you will be required to take so that you can focus your studying on those areas.

Retesting is generally permitted by HESI, but individual schools may have their own rules on the subject. Likewise, individual schools may set their own policies on whether section scores from different sessions of the HESI can be combined to get one score, or whether a score must come from one coherent session. Students with disabilities may seek accommodations from the schools administering the exam.

Test Format

The exam can include up to eight academic sections with the following distribution of questions:

Section	# of Questions
Mathematics	50
Reading Comprehension	47
Vocabulary	50
Grammar	50
Biology	25
Chemistry	25
Anatomy & Physiology	25
Physics	25

Additionally, there is a Personality Profile and Learning Style Assessment that may be included. Like the academic sections, schools can pick and choose whether to include one, both, or neither of these assessments. Each takes about 15 minutes, and you do not need to study for them.

Scoring

Prospective students and their educational institutions both receive detailed score reports after a prospective applicant completes the exam. Individual student reports include scoring explanations and breakdowns by topic for incorrect answers. The test taker's results can also include study tips based on the individual's Learning Style assessment and identification of the test taker's dominant personality type, strengths, weaknesses, and suggested learning techniques, based on the Personality Profile.

There is no set passing score for the HESI. Instead, individual schools set their own requirements and processes for incorporating scores into admissions decisions. However, HESI recommends that RN and HP programs require a 75% score to pass, and that LPN/LVN programs require a 70% score to pass.

HESI A2 Practice Test #1

Mathematics

1. Which of the following is equivalent to the value of the digit 3 in the number 792.134?
    a. 3×10
    b. 3×100
    c. $\dfrac{3}{10}$
    d. $\dfrac{3}{100}$

2. Add $101,694 + 623$.
    a. 103,317
    b. 102,317
    c. 102,417
    d. 102,427

3. How will the number 847.89632 be written if rounded to the nearest hundredth?
    a. 847.90
    b. 900
    c. 847.89
    d. 847.896

4. What is the value of the sum of $\frac{1}{3}$ and $\frac{2}{5}$?
    a. $\dfrac{3}{8}$
    b. $\dfrac{11}{15}$
    c. $\dfrac{11}{30}$
    d. $\dfrac{4}{5}$

5. Add and express in reduced form $7/12 + 5/9$.
    a. $1\dfrac{5}{36}$
    b. 13/9
    c. 41/36
    d. $1\dfrac{4}{9}$

6. How will $\frac{4}{5}$ be written as a percent?
    a. 40%
    b. 125%
    c. 90%
    d. 80%

7. Subtract 7,236 – 978.
    a. 6,268
    b. 5,258
    c. 6,358
    d. 6,258

8. What are all the factors of 12?
    a. 12, 24, 36
    b. 1, 2, 4, 6, 12
    c. 12, 24, 36, 48
    d. 1, 2, 3, 4, 6, 12

9. A construction company is building a new housing development with the property of each house measuring 30 feet wide. If the length of the street is zoned off at 345 feet, how many houses can be built on the street?
    a. 11
    b. 115
    c. 11.5
    d. 12

10. Subtract 653.4 – 59.38.
    a. 595.92
    b. 594.11
    c. 594.02
    d. 593.92

11. Subtract and express in reduced form 19/24 – 1/6.
    a. 5/8
    b. 18/6
    c. $\frac{15}{24}$
    d. 1/3

12. If $-3(x + 4) \geq x + 8$, what is the value of x?
    a. $x = 4$
    b. $x \geq 2$
    c. $x \geq -5$
    d. $x \leq -5$

13. Multiply 346×13.
    a. 4,598
    b. 4,468
    c. 4,498
    d. 4,568

14. Which inequality represents the values displayed on the number line?

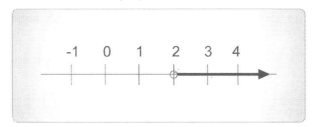

    a. $x < 2$
    b. $x \leq 2$
    c. $x > 2$
    d. $x \geq 2$

15. What is the 42nd item in the pattern: ▲○○□ ▲○○□ ▲ ...?
    a. ○
    b. ▲
    c. □
    d. None of the above

16. Which is closest to 17.8×9.9?
    a. 140
    b. 180
    c. 200
    d. 350

17. 12 is 40% of what number?
    a. 24
    b. 28
    c. 34
    d. 30

18. $3\frac{2}{3} - 1\frac{4}{5} =$

    a. $1\frac{13}{15}$

    b. $\frac{14}{15}$

    c. $2\frac{2}{3}$

    d. $\frac{4}{5}$

19. What is $\frac{660}{100}$ rounded to the nearest integer?
    a. 67
    b. 66
    c. 7
    d. 6

20. Which of the following is largest?
     a. – 0.45
     b. – 0.096
     c. – 0.3
     d. – 0.313

21. What is the value of b in this equation?

$$5b - 4 = 2b + 17$$

     a. 13
     b. 24
     c. 7
     d. 21

22. Katie works at a clothing company and sold 192 shirts over the weekend. $1/3$ of the shirts that were sold were patterned, and the rest were solid. Which mathematical expression would calculate the number of solid shirts Katie sold over the weekend?

     a. $192 \times \frac{1}{3}$

     b. $192 \div \frac{1}{3}$

     c. $192 \times (1 - \frac{1}{3})$

     d. $192 \div 3$

23. Which measure for the center of a small sample set is most affected by outliers?
     a. Mean
     b. Median
     c. Mode
     d. None of the above

24. Divide and reduce $5/13 \div 25/169$.
     a. 13/5
     b. 65/25
     c. 25/65
     d. 5/13

25. Express as a reduced mixed number 54/15.
     a. 3 3/5
     b. 3 1/15
     c. 3 3/54
     d. 3 1/54

26. in the problem $5 \times 6 + 4 \div 2 - 1$, which operation should be completed first?
     a. Multiplication
     b. Addition
     c. Division
     d. Subtraction

27. Express as an improper fraction 8 3/7.
    a. 11/7
    b. 21/8
    c. 5/3
    d. 59/7

28. Express as an improper fraction 11 5/8.
    a. 55/8
    b. 93/8
    c. 16/11
    d. 19/5

29. Round to the nearest tenth 8.067.
    a. 8.07
    b. 8.10
    c. 8.00
    d. 8.11

30. When rounding 245.2678 to the nearest thousandth, which place value would be used to decide whether to round up or round down?
    a. Ten-thousandth
    b. Thousandth
    c. Hundredth
    d. Thousand

31. Carey bought 184 pounds of fertilizer to use on her lawn. Each segment of her lawn required $12\frac{1}{2}$ pounds of fertilizer to do a sufficient job. If a student were asked to determine how many segments could be fertilized with the amount purchased, what operation would be necessary to solve this problem?
    a. Multiplication
    b. Division
    c. Addition
    d. Subtraction

32. Which of the following is an equivalent measurement for 1.3 cm?
    a. 0.13 m
    b. 0.013 m
    c. 0.13 mm
    d. 0.013 mm

33. Alan currently weighs 200 pounds, but he wants to lose weight to get down to 175 pounds. What is this difference in kilograms? (1 pound is approximately equal to 0.45 kilograms.)
    a. 9 kg
    b. 11.25 kg
    c. 78.75 kg
    d. 90 kg

34. $\frac{14}{15} + \frac{3}{5} - \frac{1}{30} =$

    a. $\frac{19}{15}$

    b. $\frac{43}{30}$

    c. $\frac{4}{3}$

    d. $\frac{3}{2}$

35. $\frac{1}{2}\sqrt{16} =$
    a. 0
    b. 1
    c. 2
    d. 4

36. Express 517 in Roman numerals.
    a. CXVII
    b. DCIIV
    c. DXVII
    d. VDVII

37. Convert 1500 hours into a 12-hour clock time.
    a. 3:00 p.m.
    b. 9:00 a.m.
    c. 3:00 a.m.
    d. 9:00 p.m.

38. $\frac{5}{3} \times \frac{7}{6} =$

    a. $\frac{3}{5}$
    b. $\frac{18}{3}$
    c. $\frac{45}{31}$
    d. $\frac{35}{18}$

39. Which common denominator would be used to evaluate $\frac{2}{3} + \frac{4}{5}$?
    a. 15
    b. 3
    c. 5
    d. 10

40. What time is 10:00am in military (24-hour clock) time?
    a. 0100 hours
    b. 1000 hours
    c. 1200 hours
    d. 0200 hours

41. 1 kilometer is how many centimeters?
    a. 100 cm
    b. 1,000 cm
    c. 10,000 cm
    d. 100,000 cm

42. What is the solution to $(2 \times 20) \div (7 + 1) + (6 \times 0.01) + (4 \times 0.001)$?
    a. 5.064
    b. 5.64
    c. 5.0064
    d. 48.064

43. $-\frac{1}{3}\sqrt{81} =$
    a. -9
    b. -3
    c. 0
    d. 3

44. A piggy bank contains 12 dollars' worth of nickels. A nickel weighs 5 grams, and the empty piggy bank weighs 1050 grams. What is the total weight of the full piggy bank?
    a. 1,110 grams
    b. 1,200 grams
    c. 2,250 grams
    d. 2,200 grams

45. Last year, the New York City area received approximately $27\frac{3}{4}$ inches of snow. The Denver area received approximately 3 times as much snow as New York City. How much snow fell in Denver?
    a. 60 inches
    b. $27\frac{1}{4}$ inches
    c. $9\frac{1}{4}$ inches
    d. $83\frac{1}{4}$ inches

46. How many pints are in 15 gallons?
    a. 45 pts.
    b. 100 pts.
    c. 120 pts.
    d. 15 pts.

47. A patient has a temperature of 37.4 °C. What is this on the Fahrenheit scale?
    a. 99.23 °F
    b. 99.32 °F
    c. 98.32 °F
    d. 98.23 °F

15

48. Dwayne has received the following scores on his math tests: 79, 91, 82, 98. What score must Dwayne get on his next math test to have an overall average of at least 90?
    a. 89
    b. 98
    c. 95
    d. 100

49. What is the overall median of Dwayne's current scores: 79, 91, 82, 98?
    a. 80.5
    b. 85
    c. 87.5
    d. 83

50. Write the expression for three times the sum of twice a number and one minus 6.
    a. $2x + 1 - 6$
    b. $3x + 1 - 6$
    c. $3(x + 1) - 6$
    d. $3(2x + 1) - 6$

Reading Comprehension

Questions 1-6 are based on the following passage:

This excerpt is an adaptation of Jonathan Swift's Gulliver's Travels into Several Remote Nations of the World.

My gentleness and good behaviour had gained so far on the emperor and his court, and indeed upon the army and people in general, that I began to conceive hopes of getting my liberty in a short time. I took all possible methods to cultivate this favourable disposition. The natives came, by degrees, to be less apprehensive of any danger from me. I would sometimes lie down, and let five or six of them dance on my hand; and at last the boys and girls would venture to come and play at hide-and-seek in my hair. I had now made a good progress in understanding and speaking the language. The emperor had a mind one day to entertain me with several of the country shows, wherein they exceed all nations I have known, both for dexterity and magnificence. I was diverted with none so much as that of the rope-dancers, performed upon a slender white thread, extended about two feet, and twelve inches from the ground. Upon which I shall desire liberty, with the reader's patience, to enlarge a little.

This diversion is only practised by those persons who are candidates for great employments, and high favour at court. They are trained in this art from their youth, and are not always of noble birth, or liberal education. When a great office is vacant, either by death or disgrace (which often happens,) five or six of those candidates petition the emperor to entertain his majesty and the court with a dance on the rope; and whoever jumps the highest, without falling, succeeds in the office. Very often the chief ministers themselves are commanded to show their skill, and to convince the emperor that they have not lost their faculty. Flimnap, the treasurer, is allowed to cut a caper on the straight rope, at least an inch higher than any other lord in the whole empire. I have seen him do the summerset several times together, upon a trencher fixed on a rope which is no thicker than a common packthread in England. My friend Reldresal, principal secretary for private affairs, is, in my opinion, if I am not partial, the second after the treasurer; the rest of the great officers are much upon a par.

1. Which of the following statements best summarize the central purpose of this text?
    a. Gulliver details his fondness for the archaic yet interesting practices of his captors.
    b. Gulliver conjectures about the intentions of the aristocratic sector of society.
    c. Gulliver becomes acquainted with the people and practices of his new surroundings.
    d. Gulliver's differences cause him to become penitent around new acquaintances.

2. What is the word *principal* referring to in the following text?
    My friend Reldresal, principal secretary for private affairs, is, in my opinion, if I am not partial, the second after the treasurer; the rest of the great officers are much upon a par.

    a. Primary or chief
    b. An acolyte
    c. An individual who provides nurturing
    d. One in a subordinate position

3. What can the reader infer from this passage?
    I would sometimes lie down, and let five or six of them dance on my hand; and at last the boys and girls would venture to come and play at hide-and-seek in my hair.

    a. The children tortured Gulliver.
    b. Gulliver traveled because he wanted to meet new people.
    c. Gulliver is considerably larger than the children who are playing around him.
    d. Gulliver has a genuine love and enthusiasm for people of all sizes.

4. What is the significance of the word *mind* in the following passage?
    The emperor had a mind one day to entertain me with several of the country shows, wherein they exceed all nations I have known, both for dexterity and magnificence.

    a. The ability to think
    b. A collective vote
    c. A definitive decision
    d. A mythological question

5. Which of the following assertions does not support the fact that games are a commonplace event in this culture?
    a. My gentlest and good behavior . . . short time.
    b. They are trained in this art from their youth . . . liberal education.
    c. Very often the chief ministers themselves are commanded to show their skill . . . not lost their faculty.
    d. Flimnap, the treasurer, is allowed to cut a caper on the straight rope . . . higher than any other lord in the whole empire.

6. How does Gulliver's description of Flimnap's, the treasurer's, ability to *cut a caper on the straight rope*, and Reldresal, principal secretary for private affairs, being the *second to the treasurer,* serve as evidence of the community's emphasis in regards to the correlation between physical strength and leadership abilities?

    a. Only children used Gulliver's hands as a playground.

    b. The two men who exhibited superior abilities held prominent positions in the community.

    c. Only common townspeople, not leaders, walk the straight rope.

    d. No one could jump higher than Gulliver.

Questions 7–9 are based on the following passage:

This excerpt is adaptation from "The 'Hatchery' of the Sun-Fish"--- *Scientific American, #711*

> I have thought that an example of the intelligence (instinct?) of a class of fish which has come under my observation during my excursions into the Adirondack region of New York State might possibly be of interest to your readers, especially as I am not aware that any one except myself has noticed it, or, at least, has given it publicity.
>
> The female sun-fish (called, I believe, in England, the roach or bream) makes a "hatchery" for her eggs in this wise. Selecting a spot near the banks of the numerous lakes in which this region abounds, and where the water is about 4 inches deep, and still, she builds, with her tail and snout, a circular embankment 3 inches in height and 2 thick. The circle, which is as perfect a one as could be formed with mathematical instruments, is usually a foot and a half in diameter; and at one side of this circular wall an opening is left by the fish of just sufficient width to admit her body.
>
> The mother sun-fish, having now built or provided her "hatchery," deposits her spawn within the circular inclosure, and mounts guard at the entrance until the fry are hatched out and are sufficiently large to take charge of themselves. As the embankment, moreover, is built up to the surface of the water, no enemy can very easily obtain an entrance within the inclosure from the top; while there being only one entrance, the fish is able, with comparative ease, to keep out all intruders.
>
> I have, as I say, noticed this beautiful instinct of the sun-fish for the perpetuity of her species more particularly in the lakes of this region; but doubtless the same habit is common to these fish in other waters.

7. What is the purpose of this passage?

    a. To show the effects of fish hatcheries on the Adirondack region

    b. To persuade the audience to study Ichthyology (fish science)

    c. To depict the sequence of mating among sun-fish

    d. To enlighten the audience on the habits of sun-fish and their hatcheries

8. How is the circle that keeps the larvae of the sun-fish made?

    a. It is formed with mathematical instruments.

    b. The sun-fish builds it with her tail and snout.

    c. It is provided to her as a "hatchery" by Mother Nature.

    d. The sun-fish builds it with her larvae.

9. The author included the third paragraph in the following passage to achieve which of the following effects?
    a. To complicate the subject matter
    b. To express a bias
    c. To insert a counterargument
    d. To conclude a sequence and add a final detail

Questions 10–14 are based on the following passage:

In the quest to understand existence, modern philosophers must question if humans can fully comprehend the world. Classical western approaches to philosophy tend to hold that one can understand something, be it an event or object, by standing outside of the phenomena and observing it. It is then by unbiased observation that one can grasp the details of the world. This seems to hold true for many things. Scientists conduct experiments and record their findings, and thus many natural phenomena become comprehendible. However, several of these observations were possible because humans used tools in order to make these discoveries.

This may seem like an extraneous matter. After all, people invented things like microscopes and telescopes in order to enhance their capacity to view cells or the movement of stars. While humans are still capable of seeing things, the question remains if human beings have the capacity to fully observe and see the world in order to understand it. It would not be an impossible stretch to argue that what humans see through a microscope is not the exact thing itself, but a human interpretation of it.

This would seem to be the case in the "Business of the Holes" experiment conducted by Richard Feynman. To study the way electrons behave, Feynman set up a barrier with two holes and a plate. The plate was there to indicate how many times the electrons would pass through the hole(s). Rather than casually observe the electrons acting under normal circumstances, Feynman discovered that electrons behave in two totally different ways depending on whether or not they are observed. The electrons that were observed had passed through either one of the holes or were caught on the plate as particles. However, electrons that weren't observed acted as waves instead of particles and passed through both holes. This indicated that electrons have a dual nature. Electrons seen by the human eye act like particles, while unseen electrons act like waves of energy.

This dual nature of the electrons presents a conundrum. While humans now have a better understanding of electrons, the fact remains that people cannot entirely perceive how electrons behave without the use of instruments. We can only observe one of the mentioned behaviors, which only provides a partial understanding of the entire function of electrons. Therefore, we're forced to ask ourselves whether the world we observe is objective or if it is subjectively perceived by humans. Or, an alternative question: can man understand the world only through machines that will allow them to observe natural phenomena?

Both questions humble man's capacity to grasp the world. However, those ideas don't take into account that many phenomena have been proven by human beings without the use of machines, such as the discovery of gravity. Like all philosophical questions, whether man's

19

reason and observation alone can understand the universe can be approached from many angles.

10. The word *extraneous* in paragraph two can be best interpreted as referring to which one of the following?
   a. Indispensable
   b. Bewildering
   c. Superfluous
   d. Exuberant

11. What is the author's motivation for writing the passage?
   a. Bring to light an alternative view on human perception by examining the role of technology in human understanding.
   b. Educate the reader on the latest astroparticle physics discovery and offer terms that may be unfamiliar to the reader.
   c. Argue that humans are totally blind to the realities of the world by presenting an experiment that proves that electrons are not what they seem on the surface.
   d. Reflect on opposing views of human understanding.

12. Which of the following most closely resembles the way in which paragraph four is structured?
   a. It offers one solution, questions the solution, and then ends with an alternative solution.
   b. It presents an inquiry, explains the detail of that inquiry, and then offers a solution.
   c. It presents a problem, explains the details of that problem, and then ends with more inquiry.
   d. It gives a definition, offers an explanation, and then ends with an inquiry.

13. For the classical approach to understanding to hold true, which of the following must be required?
   a. A telescope.
   b. The person observing must prove their theory beyond a doubt.
   c. Multiple witnesses present.
   d. The person observing must be unbiased.

14. Which best describes how the electrons in the experiment behaved like waves?
   a. The electrons moved up and down like actual waves.
   b. The electrons passed through both holes and then onto the plate.
   c. The electrons converted to photons upon touching the plate.
   d. Electrons were seen passing through one hole or the other.

Questions 15-20 are based on the following passage:

The Middle Ages were a time of great superstition and theological debate. Many beliefs were developed and practiced, while some died out or were listed as heresy. Boethianism is a Medieval theological philosophy that attributes sin to gratification and righteousness with virtue and God's providence. Boethianism holds that sin, greed, and corruption are means to attain temporary pleasure, but that they inherently harm the person's soul as well as other human beings.

In *The Canterbury Tales,* we observe more instances of bad actions punished than goodness being rewarded. This would appear to be some reflection of Boethianism. In the "Pardoner's Tale," all three thieves wind up dead, which is a result of their desire for wealth. Each wrong doer pays with their life, and they are unable to enjoy the wealth they worked to steal. Within his tales, Chaucer gives reprieve to people undergoing struggle, but also interweaves stories of contemptible individuals being cosmically punished for their wickedness. The thieves idolize physical wealth, which leads to their downfall. This same theme and ideological principle of Boethianism is repeated in the "Friar's Tale," whose summoner character attempts to gain further wealth by partnering with a demon. The summoner's refusal to repent for his avarice and corruption leads to the demon dragging his soul to Hell. Again, we see the theme of the individual who puts faith and morality aside in favor for a physical prize. The result, of course, is that the summoner loses everything.

The examples of the righteous being rewarded tend to appear in a spiritual context within the *Canterbury Tales*. However, there are a few instances where we see goodness resulting in physical reward. In the Prioress' Tale, we see corporal punishment for barbarism *and* a reward for goodness. The Jews are punished for their murder of the child, giving a sense of law and order (though racist) to the plot. While the boy does die, he is granted a lasting reward by being able to sing even after his death, a miracle that marks that the murdered youth led a pure life. Here, the miracle represents eternal favor with God.

Again, we see the theological philosophy of Boethianism in Chaucer's *The Canterbury Tales* through acts of sin and righteousness and the consequences that follow. When pleasures of the world are sought instead of God's favor, we see characters being punished in tragic ways. However, the absence of worldly lust has its own set of consequences for the characters seeking to obtain God's favor.

15. What would be a potential reward for living a good life, as described in Boethianism?
    a. A long life sustained by the good deeds one has done over a lifetime
    b. Wealth and fertility for oneself and the extension of one's family line
    c. Vengeance for those who have been persecuted by others who have a capacity for committing wrongdoing
    d. God's divine favor for one's righteousness

16. What might be the main reason why the author chose to discuss Boethianism through examining The Canterbury Tales?
    a. *The Canterbury Tales* is a well-known text.
    b. *The Canterbury Tales* is the only known fictional text that contains use of Boethianism.
    c. *The Canterbury Tales* presents a manuscript written in the medieval period that can help illustrate Boethianism through stories and show how people of the time might have responded to the idea.
    d. Within each individual tale in *The Canterbury Tales*, the reader can read about different levels of Boethianism and how each level leads to greater enlightenment.

17. What "ideological principle" is the author referring to in the middle of the second paragraph when talking about the "Friar's Tale"?
    a. The principle that the act of ravaging another's possessions is the same as ravaging one's soul.
    b. The principle that thieves who idolize physical wealth will be punished in an earthly sense as well as eternally.
    c. The principle that fraternization with a demon will result in one losing everything, including his or her life.
    d. The principle that a desire for material goods leads to moral malfeasance punishable by a higher being.

18. Which of the following words, if substituted for the word *avarice* in paragraph two, would LEAST change the meaning of the sentence?
    a. Perniciousness
    b. Pithiness
    c. Parsimoniousness
    d. Precariousness

19. Based on the passage, what view does Boethianism take on desire?
    a. Desire does not exist in the context of Boethianism
    b. Desire is a virtue and should be welcomed
    c. Having desire is evidence of demonic possession
    d. Desire for pleasure can lead toward sin

Questions 20-25 are based on the following, which is an excerpt is an adaptation of Robert Louis Stevenson's The Strange Case of Dr. Jekyll and Mr. Hyde.

"Did you ever come across a protégé of his—one Hyde?" He asked.

"Hyde?" repeated Lanyon. "No. Never heard of him. Since my time."

That was the amount of information that the lawyer carried back with him to the great, dark bed on which he tossed to and fro until the small hours of the morning began to grow large. It was a night of little ease to his toiling mind, toiling in mere darkness and besieged by questions.

Six o'clock struck on the bells of the church that was so conveniently near to Mr. Utterson's dwelling, and still he was digging at the problem. Hitherto it had touched him on the intellectual side alone; but; but now his imagination also was engaged, or rather enslaved; and as he lay and tossed in the gross darkness of the night in the curtained room, Mr. Enfield's tale went by before his mind in a scroll of lighted pictures. He would be aware of the great field of lamps in a nocturnal city; then of the figure of a man walking swiftly; then of a child running from the doctor's; and then these met, and that human Juggernaut trod the child down and passed on regardless of her screams. Or else he would see a room in a rich house, where his friend lay asleep, dreaming and smiling at his dreams; and then the door of that room would be opened, the curtains of the bed plucked apart, the sleeper recalled, and, lo! There would stand by his side a figure to whom power was given, and even at that dead hour he must rise and do its bidding. The figure in these two phrases haunted the lawyer all night; and if at anytime he dozed over, it was but to see it glide more stealthily through sleeping houses, or move the more swiftly, and still the more smoothly, even to dizziness, through wider labyrinths of lamplighted city, and at every street corner crush a child and leave her screaming. And still the figure had no face by which he might know it; even in his dreams it had no face, or one that baffled him and melted before his eyes; and thus there it was that there sprung up and grew apace in the lawyer's mind a singularly strong, almost an inordinate, curiosity to behold the features of the real Mr. Hyde. If he could but once set eyes on him, he thought the mystery would lighten and perhaps roll altogether away, as was the habit of mysterious things when well examined. He might see a reason for his friend's strange preference or bondage, and even for the startling clauses of the will. And at least it would be a face worth seeing: the face of a man who was without bowels of mercy: a face which had but to show itself to raise up, in the mind of the unimpressionable Enfield, a spirit of enduring hatred.

From that time forward, Mr. Utterson began to haunt the door in the by street of shops. In the morning before office hours, at noon when business was plenty of time scares, at night under the face of the full city moon, by all lights and at all hours of solitude or concourse, the lawyer was to be found on his chosen post.

"If he be Mr. Hyde," he had thought, "I should be Mr. Seek."

20. What is the purpose of the use of repetition in the following passage?
    It was a night of little ease to his toiling mind, toiling in mere darkness and besieged by questions.

    a. It serves as a demonstration of the mental state of Mr. Lanyon.
    b. It is reminiscent of the church bells that are mentioned in the story.
    c. It mimics Mr. Utterson's ambivalence.
    d. It emphasizes Mr. Utterson's anguish in failing to identify Hyde's whereabouts.

21. What is the setting of the story in this passage?
    a. In the city
    b. On the countryside
    c. In a jail
    d. In a mental health facility

22. What can one infer about the meaning of the word "Juggernaut" from the author's use of it in the passage?
    a. It is an apparition that appears at daybreak.
    b. It scares children.
    c. It is associated with space travel.
    d. Mr. Utterson finds it soothing.

23. What is the definition of the word *haunt* in the following passage?

> From that time forward, Mr. Utterson began to haunt the door in the by street of shops. In the morning before office hours, at noon when business was plenty of time scares, at night under the face of the full city moon, by all lights and at all hours of solitude or concourse, the lawyer was to be found on his chosen post.

    a. To levitate
    b. To constantly visit
    c. To terrorize
    d. To daunt

24. The phrase *labyrinths of lamplighted city* contains an example of what?
    a. Hyperbole
    b. Simile
    c. Metaphor
    d. Alliteration

25. What can one reasonably conclude from the final comment of this passage?

> "If he be Mr. Hyde," he had thought, "I should be Mr. Seek."

    a. The speaker is considering a name change.
    b. The speaker is experiencing an identity crisis.
    c. The speaker has mistakenly been looking for the wrong person.
    d. The speaker intends to continue to look for Hyde.

Questions 26–31 are based upon the following passage:

This excerpt is adaptation from *Our Vanishing Wildlife,* by William T. Hornaday

> Three years ago, I think there were not many bird-lovers in the United States, who believed it possible to prevent the total extinction of both egrets from our fauna. All the known rookeries accessible to plume-hunters had been totally destroyed. Two years ago, the secret discovery of several small, hidden colonies prompted William Dutcher, President of the National Association of Audubon Societies, and Mr. T. Gilbert Pearson, Secretary, to attempt the protection of those colonies. With a fund contributed for the purpose, wardens were hired and duly commissioned. As previously stated, one of those wardens was shot dead in cold blood by a plume hunter. The task of guarding swamp rookeries from the attacks of money-hungry desperadoes to whom the accursed plumes were worth their weight in gold, is a very chancy proceeding. There is now one warden in Florida who says that "before they get my rookery they will first have to get me."

> Thus far the protective work of the Audubon Association has been successful. Now there are twenty colonies, which contain all told, about 5,000 egrets and about 120,000 herons and ibises which are guarded by the Audubon wardens. One of the most important is on Bird Island, a mile out in Orange Lake, central Florida, and it is ably defended by Oscar E. Baynard. To-day, the plume hunters who do not dare to raid the guarded rookeries are trying to study out the lines of flight of the birds, to and from their feeding-grounds, and shoot them in transit. Their motto is—"Anything to beat the law, and get the plumes." It is there that the state of Florida should take part in the war.

The success of this campaign is attested by the fact that last year a number of egrets were seen in eastern Massachusetts—for the first time in many years. And so to-day the question is, can the wardens continue to hold the plume-hunters at bay?

26. The author's use of first person pronoun in the following text does NOT have which of the following effects?

> Three years ago, I think there were not many bird-lovers in the United States, who believed it possible to prevent the total extinction of both egrets from our fauna.

    a. The phrase *I think* acts as a sort of hedging, where the author's tone is less direct and/or absolute.
    b. It allows the reader to more easily connect with the author.
    c. It encourages the reader to empathize with the egrets.
    d. It distances the reader from the text by overemphasizing the story.

27. What purpose does the quote serve at the end of the first paragraph?
    a. The quote shows proof of a hunter threatening one of the wardens.
    b. The quote lightens the mood by illustrating the colloquial language of the region.
    c. The quote provides an example of a warden protecting one of the colonies.
    d. The quote provides much needed comic relief in the form of a joke.

28. What is the meaning of the word *rookeries* in the following text?

> To-day, the plume hunters who do not dare to raid the guarded rookeries are trying to study out the lines of flight of the birds, to and from their feeding-grounds, and shoot them in transit.

    a. Houses in a slum area
    b. A place where hunters gather to trade tools
    c. A place where wardens go to trade stories
    d. A colony of breeding birds

29. What is on Bird Island?
    a. Hunters selling plumes
    b. An important bird colony
    c. Bird Island Battle between the hunters and the wardens
    d. An important egret with unique plumes

30. What is the main purpose of the passage?
    a. To persuade the audience to act in preservation of the bird colonies
    b. To show the effect hunting egrets has had on the environment
    c. To argue that the preservation of bird colonies has had a negative impact on the environment.
    d. To demonstrate the success of the protective work of the Audubon Association

31. Why are hunters trying to study the lines of flight of the birds?
    a. To study ornithology, one must know the lines of flight that birds take.
    b. To help wardens preserve the lives of the birds
    c. To have a better opportunity to hunt the birds
    d. To builds their homes under the lines of flight because they believe it brings good luck

Read the following poem and answer questions 32–37:

Two roads diverged in a yellow wood,
And sorry I could not travel both
And be one traveler, long I stood
And looked down one as far as I could
To where it bent in the undergrowth;   5
Then took the other, as just as fair,
And having perhaps the better claim,
Because it was grassy and wanted wear;
Though as for that the passing there
Had worn them really about the same,   10
And both that morning equally lay
In leaves no step had trodden black.
Oh, I kept the first for another day!
Yet knowing how way leads on to way,
I doubted if I should ever come back.   15
I shall be telling this with a sigh
Somewhere ages and ages hence:
Two roads diverged in a wood, and I—
I took the one less traveled by,
And that has made all the difference.   20

Robert Frost, "The Road Not Taken"

32. Which option best expresses the symbolic meaning of the "road" and the overall theme?
    a. A divergent spot where the traveler had to choose the correct path to his destination
    b. A choice between good and evil that the traveler needs to make
    c. The traveler's struggle between his lost love and his future prospects
    d. Life's journey and the choices with which humans are faced

33. How many lines are there in this poem?
    a. 10
    b. 15
    c. 20
    d. 21

34. How many stanzas are there in this poem?
    a. 1
    b. 2
    c. 3
    d. 4

35. How many travelers are there in the poem?
    a. 1
    b. 2
    c. 3
    d. 4

36. What is the time of day in the poem?
    a. Night
    b. Morning
    c. Evening
    d. Afternoon

37. Which road did the traveler take?
    a. The first
    b. The second
    c. Both
    d. Neither

38. Which option best exemplifies an author's use of alliteration and personification?
    a. Her mood hung about her like a weary cape, very dull from wear.
    b. It shuddered, swayed, shook, and screamed its way into dust under hot flames.
    c. The house was a starch sentry, warning visitors away.
    d. At its shoreline, visitors swore they heard the siren call of the cliffs above.

39. In 1889, Jerome K. Jerome wrote a humorous account of a boating holiday. Originally intended as a chapter in a serious travel guide, the work became a prime example of a comic novel. Read the passage below, noting the word/words in italics. Answer the question that follows.

> I felt rather hurt about this at first; it seemed somehow to be a sort of slight. Why hadn't I got housemaid's knee? Why this invidious reservation? After a while, however, less grasping feelings prevailed. I reflected that I had every other known malady in the pharmacology, and I grew less selfish, and determined to do without housemaid's knee. Gout, in its most malignant stage, it would appear, had seized me without my being aware of it; and *zymosis* I had evidently been suffering with from boyhood. There were no more diseases after *zymosis*, so I concluded there was nothing else the matter with me. —Jerome K. Jerome, *Three Men in a Boat*

Which definition best fits the word *zymosis*?
    a. Discontent
    b. An infectious disease
    c. Poverty
    d. Bad luck

40. What is the meaning of the word *rookeries* in the following text?
    To-day, the plume hunters who do not dare to raid the guarded rookeries are trying to study out the lines of flight of the birds, to and from their feeding-grounds, and shoot them in transit.

    a. Houses in a slum area
    b. A place where hunters gather to trade tools
    c. A place where wardens go to trade stories
    d. A colony of breeding birds

Use the passage below for questions 41 through 42:

Caribbean Island Destinations

Do you want to vacation at a Caribbean island destination? Who wouldn't want a tropical vacation? Visit one of the many Caribbean islands where visitors can swim in crystal blue waters, swim with dolphins, or enjoy family-friendly or adult-only resorts and activities. Every island offers a unique and picturesque vacation destination. Choose from these islands: Aruba, St. Lucia, Barbados, Anguilla, St. John, and so many more. A Caribbean island destination will be the best and most refreshing vacation ever . . . no regrets!

41. What is the topic of the passage?
    a. Caribbean island destinations
    b. Tropical vacation
    c. Resorts
    d. Activities

42. What is/are the supporting detail(s) of this passage?
    a. Cruising to the Caribbean
    b. Local events
    c. Family or adult-only resorts and activities
    d. All of the above

Questions 43–48 are based on the following poem, "To Waken an Old Lady" by William Carlos Williams:

> Old age is
> a flight of small
> cheeping birds
> skimming
> bare trees   5
> above a snow glaze.
> Gaining and failing
> they are buffeted
> by a dark wind—
> But what?   10
> On harsh weedstalks
> the flock has rested,
> the snow
> is covered with broken
> seedhusks   15
> and the wind tempered
> by a shrill
> piping of plenty.

43. This poem uses which of the following literary techniques typical of its time period?
    a. Meter
    b. Anaphora
    c. Imagery
    d. Synecdoche

44. This poem comes out of which of the following literary periods?
   a. Romanticism
   b. Modernism
   c. Postmodernism
   d. Confessional poetry

45. Which of the following provides the best analysis of the poem?
   a. The poem acts as an extended metaphor of old age. Its juxtaposed imagery suggests the frailty of life ("Gaining and failing / they are buffeted / by a dark wind") alongside the fullness of life and its "piping of plenty."
   b. The poem describes a flock of birds and their relationship with nature. They rest "On harsh weedstalks" and are "buffeted / by a dark wind." The poem concludes suggesting that their greatest joy as well as their greatest strife is nature itself.
   c. The poem is an ode to the wind. Although the poem starts off comparing old age to birds, we see the poem calling upon the wind at the end in order to make sense of the world. The wind is ultimately in control in the poem—it is the driving force of the poem.
   d. This poem is about writing poetry. Old age signifies the poet, while the "small / cheeping birds" signifies the poet's words. The conclusion of the poem describes the wind as the creative process of writing a poem, and the "piping of plenty" is what the author gets in writing a fulfilling, lengthy poem.

46. What rhetorical device is shown in the very last line?
   a. Metaphor
   b. Simile
   c. Anaphora
   d. Alliteration

47. What time of year is the poem describing?
   a. Summer
   b. Fall
   c. Winter
   d. Spring

48. In the poem, what do the birds finally rest on?
   a. Seedhusks
   b. Weedstalks
   c. Trees
   d. The bare ground

Vocabulary

1. What are the blood vessels called that carry deoxygenated blood back to the heart?
   a. Capillaries
   b. Arteries
   c. Ventricles
   d. Veins

2. A patient has been vocal in the past about not needing to change anything about his lifestyle. The patient feels angry and frustrated by his conversation with the doctor. The patient is very agitated when the nurse aide comes to collect vital signs and tells her that he thinks she is lazy. What kind of defense mechanism is the patient displaying?
   a. Intellectualization
   b. Undoing
   c. Reaction formation
   d. Displacement

3. What word is a synonym for *instructor*?
   a. Pupil
   b. Teacher
   c. Survivor
   d. Dictator

4. The nurse aide walks into the room where the patient is clutching his chest, sweating, and appears short of breath. He reports that he is experiencing chest pain that is crushing and severe, with some pain in his left arm as well. Which type of chest pain is this most likely associated with?
   a. Myocardial infarction
   b. Gastroesophageal reflux
   c. Pneumonia
   d. Pleuritis

5. Which of the following is the best definition of *reconnaissance?*
   a. Preliminary surveying
   b. Capturing
   c. Proliferation and growth
   d. Ingenuity

6. What does *ineffable* mean?
   a. Insincere
   b. Inefficient
   c. Indescribable
   d. Inexperienced

7. What does *gregarious* most nearly mean?
   a. Monstrous
   b. Meek
   c. Sociable
   d. Impressive

8. What word is a synonym for *caustic*?
   a. Sarcastic
   b. Luxurious
   c. Expensive
   d. Uncooperative

9. The patient violently convulses with rigid muscles. The patient is completely unconscious. What kind of seizure is this?
    a. Myoclonic
    b. Absence
    c. Grand Mal
    d. Tonic

10. The patient is having trouble forming thoughts into sentences, and one side of his face appears to be drooping. What emergency condition is likely occurring in the patient?
    a. Meningitis
    b. Migraine
    c. Seizure
    d. Cerebrovascular accident

11. A patient with diabetes has been off the floor all morning for a test and returns just as the lunch trays are being picked up. The patient was NPO for their test so did not receive his breakfast either. What does the nurse notice this patient is at risk for?
    a. Hypoglycemia
    b. Diabetic ketoacidosis
    c. Diabetic coma
    d. Hyperglycemia

12. What is a synonym for *obtuse*?
    a. Slow-witted
    b. Large
    c. Gluttonous
    d. Stretched

13. If a patient can be described as "sleepy" yet able to be aroused by verbal stimuli, what is the term for this altered level of consciousness?
    a. Coma
    b. Delirium
    c. Somnolent
    d. Stupor

14. A patient who has been admitted with tuberculosis begins to cough up blood in their sputum. What is the medical term for this condition?
    a. Hematopoiesis
    b. Hemoptysis
    c. Hematemesis
    d. Hematochezia

15. What word means *sordid*?
    a. Semantic
    b. Surly
    c. Vile
    d. Basic

16. _____ may present with vague signs which may mimic chest pain, depression, or other physical illnesses.
    a. Bereavement
    b. Stroke
    c. Anorexia Nervosa
    d. Myocardial Infarction

17. _____ have a side effect causing excessive thirst.
    a. Antidepressants
    b. Antibiotics
    c. Antispasmodics
    d. Anti-inflammatories

18. What does *solicit* mean?
    a. Ask
    b. Donate
    c. Perturb
    d. Solace

19. What kind of ulcer is most commonly found between the knees and ankles?
    a. Arterial
    b. Neuropathic
    c. Venous
    d. Stage IV

20. What type of strength exercise is performed without moving the joint using resistance?
    a. Isometric
    b. Isotonic
    c. Isokinetic
    d. Plyometric

21. Tendons connect what?
    a. Muscle to muscle
    b. Bone to bone
    c. Muscle to bone
    d. Muscle to ligament

22. Which of the following is NOT a bone of the axial skeleton?
    a. Sternum
    b. Mandible
    c. Ilium
    d. Atlas

23. Using anatomical terms, what is the relationship of the sternum relative to the deltoid?
    a. Medial
    b. Lateral
    c. Superficial
    d. Posterior

24. The epidermis is composed of what type of cells?
    a. Osteoclasts
    b. Connective
    c. Dendritic
    d. Epithelial

25. What is the primary function of Volkmann's canals?
    a. To deliver materials from the central canal to peripheral osteocytes
    b. To strengthen the bony matrix by running parallel to the long axis of the bone
    c. To serve as the primary site where osteocytes are embedded within the bone by surrounding the Haversian canal in concentric circles
    d. To produce yellow and red bone marrow

26. The term *cubital* refers to what body region?
    a. The skin
    b. The fingertips
    c. The elbow
    d. The shoulder

27. Eosinophils are best described as which of the following?
    a. A type of granulocyte that secretes histamine, which stimulates the inflammatory response.
    b. The most abundant type of white blood cell that secretes substances that are toxic to pathogens.
    c. A type of granulocyte found under mucous membranes that defends against multicellular parasites.
    d. A type of circulating granulocyte that is aggressive and has high phagocytic activity.

28. _____ is a structural protein and the primary constituent of things like hair and nails.
    a. Keratin
    b. Antigens
    c. Channel proteins
    d. Actin

29. Which of the available words best fits in the following sentence? The dermis is _____ relative to the epidermis.
    a. Superficial
    b. Deep
    c. Superior
    d. Inferior

30. Select the correct meaning of the underlined word in the following sentence. The student wanted to become a phlebotomist.
    a. A professional who takes x-rays
    b. A professional who makes artificial limbs
    c. A professional who draws blood
    d. A professional who counsels patients

31. What word meaning "to return to an earlier state" best fits in the following sentence? The child seemed to emotionally _____ when he felt sick.

    a. Rescind

    b. Digress

    c. Regress

    d. Diverge

32. Where is the acromion process located?

    a. The spine

    b. The skull

    c. The shoulder

    d. The sternum

33. Select the correct meaning of the underlined word in the following sentence. The patient's eyes appeared glassy.

    a. Sad

    b. Expressionless

    c. Emotional

    d. Blind

34. What word meaning "to be in alignment such that there is a continuous plane" best fits in the following sentence? It is important that the brace remains _____ with the skin to avoid skin irritation.

    a. Flush

    b. Flesh

    c. Articulated

    d. Adjacent

35. What is the meaning of the word *innervate*?

    a. To attach a muscle to a bone

    b. To shorten a muscle

    c. To supply nerves to

    d. To conduct a nerve impulse

36. What is a potential complication of gangrene?

    a. Amputation

    b. Ulcer

    c. Parasites

    d. Diabetes

37. What word meaning "urgent" best fits in the following sentence? The _____ demands of the supervising physician made it difficult to complete paperwork in a timely manner.

    a. Lenient

    b. Extoll

    c. Exigent

    d. Lackadaisical

38. Select the correct meaning of the underlined word in the following sentence. The patient had aphasia after his stroke.
    a. Memory loss
    b. Droopy face
    c. Impairment in facial recognition
    d. Language impairment

39. What does the abbreviation NPO mean?
    a. Not per orders
    b. Do not resuscitate
    c. Nothing by mouth
    d. Nothing by orders

40. Select the correct meaning of the underlined word in the following sentence. The professor was notorious for his jejune lectures.
    a. Dull
    b. Stimulating
    c. Interactive
    d. Expert

41. What word meaning "shortage" best fits in the following sentence? The salary hike for all unionized workers increased the hospital's budgetary _____.
    a. Deficit
    b. Diffident
    c. Dearth
    d. Defiant

42. What is the best definition of the word *paradox*?
    a. Sensation
    b. Hypothesis
    c. Insinuation
    d. Contradiction

43. What word meaning "agile" best fits in the following sentence? The _____ dancer was graceful and beautiful to watch.
    a. Lithe
    b. Ballerina
    c. Unwieldly
    d. Chivalrous

44. What word meaning "a bluish discoloration of the skin caused by lack of oxygen" best fits in the following sentence? It is not uncommon for a chocking or drowning child to exhibit _____.
    a. Flushing
    b. Cyanosis
    c. Listless
    d. Rall

45. What is the best definition of the word *venerate*?
   a. Respect
   b. Reject
   c. Expect
   d. Deserve

46. What word meaning "a fungal infection or disease" best fits in the following sentence. Ringworm is considered a type of _____.
   a. Lichen
   b. Mycosis
   c. Virus
   d. Pustule

47. What word meaning "blood in the urine" best fits in the following sentence? A common sign of a kidney infection is _____.
   a. Anuria
   b. Nocturia
   c. Uremia
   d. Polyurea

48. What is the best definition of the word *tetanus*?
   a. A muscle twitch
   b. A sustained muscle contraction
   c. A muscle spasm
   d. Muscle paralysis

49. Select the correct meaning of the underlined word in the following sentence. The patient had a difficulty with proprioception.
   a. Spatial awareness of the body
   b. Balance and agility
   c. Pain detection
   d. Sensory integration

50. What does *abstain* mean?
   a. To regurgitate
   b. To imbibe
   c. To refrain from something
   d. To prolong

Grammar

1. Identify the noun clause in the following sentence.
   The belief that there is an afterlife is a personal choice.
   a. the belief that
   b. is a personal choice
   c. that there is an afterlife
   d. is an afterlife

2. Identify the adjective clause in the following sentence.

A boy who loves to ride bikes gets plenty of exercise.

a. a boy who loves
b. who loves to ride bikes
c. to ride bikes
d. gets plenty of exercise

3. Identify the adverbial clause in the following sentence.

I want to work in the garden longer unless you are too tired.

a. I want to work in the garden
b. in the garden
c. are too tired
d. unless you are too tired

4. Identify the noun phrase in the following sentence.

The actor and actress rode in the long black limousine.

a. actor and actress
b. rode in the
c. the long black limousine
d. actress rode in

5. Armani got lost when she walked around Paris.

Rewrite, beginning with: <u>Walking through Paris,</u>

The next words will be
a. you can get lost.
b. Armani found herself lost.
c. she should have gotten lost.
d. is about getting lost.

6. Which sentence does NOT include a gerund phrase?
a. Swimming several laps is a great way to get exercise.
b. The best way to swim quickly is using the flippers.
c. I can swim farther than the coach can in three minutes.
d. Learning to swim is not as difficult as you imagine it to be.

7. Which of the following sentences includes a nonessential appositive phrase?
a. Carrie Fisher, my second cousin, was an actress in the movie *Star Wars*.
b. The actor Harrison Ford also plays a lead role in *Star Wars*.
c. The movie *Star Wars* is about two hours long.
d. The movie *Star Wars* has become legendary.

8. Which of the following sentences highlights an absolute phrase?
a. One of my favorite activities is <u>going camping in the forest</u>.
b. <u>The fire crackling</u>, it is so exciting to be enveloped in nature.
c. The best drinks, <u>hot cocoa and coffee</u>, are served at campfires.
d. I love camping because it is the best experience <u>for school-age children</u>.

9. After his cat died, Phoenix buried the cat with her favorite toys in his backyard.

Rewrite, beginning with: <u>Phoenix buried his cat</u>

The next words will be
    a. in his backyard before she died.
    b. after she died in the backyard.
    c. with her favorite toys after she died.
    d. after he buried her toys in the backyard.

10. While I was in the helicopter I saw the sunset, and tears streamed down my eyes.

Rewrite, beginning with: <u>Tears streamed down my eyes</u>

The next words will be:
    a. while I watched the helicopter fly into the sunset.
    b. because the sunset flew up into the sky.
    c. because the helicopter was facing the sunset.
    d. when I saw the sunset from the helicopter.

For the next two questions, select the answer choice that best corrects the underlined portion of the sentence:

11. It is necessary for instructors to offer tutoring <u>to any students who need extra help in the class.</u>
    a. to any students who need extra help in the class.
    b. for any students that need extra help in the class.
    c. with any students who need extra help in the class.
    d. for any students needing any extra help in their class.

12. <u>Because many people</u> feel there are too many distractions to get any work done, I actually enjoy working from home.
    a. Because many people
    b. While many people
    c. Maybe many people
    d. With most people

Directions for questions 13-14: Rewrite the sentence in your head following the directions given below. Keep in mind that your new sentence should be well written and should have essentially the same meaning as the original sentence.

13. Student loan debt is at an all-time high, which is why many politicians are using this issue to gain the attention and votes of students, or anyone with student loan debt.

Rewrite, beginning with <u>Student loan debt is at an all-time high.</u>

The next words will be which of the following?
    a. because politicians want students' votes.
    b. , so politicians are using the issue to gain votes.
    c. , so voters are choosing politicians who care about this issue.
    d. , and politicians want to do something about it.

14. Seasoned runners often advise new runners to get fitted for better quality running shoes because new runners often complain about minor injuries like sore knees or shin splints.

Rewrite, beginning with <u>Seasoned runners often advise new runners to get fitted for better quality running shoes.</u>

The next words will be which of the following?
    a. to help them avoid minor injuries.
    b. because they know better.
    c. , so they can run further.
    d. to complain about running injuries.

15. Which sentence shows grammatically correct parallelism?
    a. The puppies enjoy chewing and to play tug-o-war.
    b. The puppies enjoy to chew and playing tug-o-war.
    c. The puppies enjoy to chew and to play tug-o-war.
    d. The puppies enjoy chewing and playing tug-o-war.

16. Which sentence shows grammatically correct parallelism?
    a. He is the clown who inflated balloons and honked his nose.
    b. He is the clown who inflated balloons and who honked his nose.
    c. He is the clown that inflated balloons and who honked his nose.
    d. He is the clown that inflated balloons and that honked his nose.

17. Which sentence shows grammatically correct parallelism?
    a. My grandparents have been traveling and have been sightseeing.
    b. My grandparents have been traveling and were sightseeing.
    c. My grandparents were traveling and have been sightseeing.
    d. My grandparents have been traveling and they're sightseeing.

18. Which sentence shows grammatically correct subordination?
    a. The building was sturdy and solid; it crumbled during the earthquake.
    b. The building was study and solid although it crumbled during the earthquake.
    c. Although the building was sturdy and solid, it crumbled during the earthquake.
    d. Despite being sturdy and solid, the building crumbled during the earthquake.

19. Which of the following examples uses correct punctuation?
    a. Recommended supplies for the hunting trip include the following: rain gear, large backpack, hiking boots, flashlight, and non-perishable foods.
    b. I left the store, because I forgot my wallet.
    c. As soon as the team checked into the hotel; they met in the lobby for a group photo.
    d. None of the furniture came in on time: so they weren't able to move in to the new apartment.

20. Which of the following sentences shows correct word usage?
    a. Your going to have to put you're jacket over their.
    b. You're going to have to put your jacket over there.
    c. Your going to have to put you're jacket over they're.
    d. You're going to have to put you're jacket over their.

21. A student wants to rewrite the following sentence:
    Entrepreneurs use their ideas to make money.

He wants to use the word *money* as a verb, but he isn't sure which word ending to use. What is the appropriate suffix to add to *money* to complete the following sentence?

Entrepreneurs _____ their ideas.

    a. –ize
    b. –ical
    c. –en
    d. –ful

22. Which of the following sentences has an error in capitalization?
    a. The East Coast has experienced very unpredictable weather this year.
    b. My Uncle owns a home in Florida, where he lives in the winter.
    c. I am taking English Composition II on campus this fall.
    d. There are several nice beaches we can visit on our trip to the Jersey Shore this summer.

23. Julia Robinson, an avid photographer in her spare time, was able to capture stunning shots of the local wildlife on her last business trip to Australia.
Which of the following is an adjective in the preceding sentence?
    a. Time
    b. Capture
    c. Avid
    d. Photographer

24. Which of the following sentences uses correct punctuation?
    a. Carole is not currently working; her focus is on her children at the moment.
    b. Carole is not currently working and her focus is on her children at the moment.
    c. Carole is not currently working, her focus is on her children at the moment.
    d. Carole is not currently working her focus is on her children at the moment.

25. Which of these examples is a compound sentence?
    a. Alex and Shane spent the morning coloring and later took a walk down to the park.
    b. After coloring all morning, Alex and Shane spent the afternoon at the park.
    c. Alex and Shane spent the morning coloring, and then they took a walk down to the park.
    d. After coloring all morning and spending part of the day at the park, Alex and Shane took a nap.

26. Glorify, fortify, gentrify, acidify

Based on the preceding words, what is the correct meaning of the suffix *–fy*?
    a. Marked by, given to
    b. Doer, believer
    c. Make, cause, cause to have
    d. Process, state, rank

27. After a long day at work, Tracy had dinner with her family, and then took a walk to the park. What are the transitional words in the preceding sentence?
    a. After, then
    b. At, with, to
    c. Had, took
    d. A, the

28. Which of the following examples is a compound sentence?
    a. Shawn and Jerome played soccer in the backyard for two hours.
    b. Marissa last saw Elena and talked to her this morning.
    c. The baby was sick, so I decided to stay home from work.
    d. Denise, Kurt, and Eric went for a run after dinner.

29. Robert needed to find at least four sources for his final project, so he searched several library databases for reliable academic research. Which words function as nouns in the preceding sentence?
    a. Robert, sources, project, databases, research
    b. Robert, sources, final, project, databases, academic, research
    c. Robert, sources, project, he, library, databases, research
    d. Sources, project, databases, research

30. Which of the following sentences uses correct subject-verb agreement?
    a. There is two constellations that can be seen from the back of the house.
    b. At least four of the sheep needs to be sheared before the end of summer.
    c. Lots of people were auditioning for the singing competition on Saturday.
    d. Everyone in the group have completed the assignment on time.

31. Philadelphia is home to some excellent walking tours where visitors can learn more about the culture and rich history of the city of brotherly love. What are the adjectives in the preceding sentence?
    a. Philadelphia, tours, visitors, culture, history, city, love
    b. Excellent, walking, rich, brotherly
    c. Is, can, learn
    d. To, about, of

32. Which sentence has a misplaced modifier?
    a. The children love their cute and cuddly teddy bears.
    b. Teddy bears are cute and cuddly; the children love them.
    c. Cute and cuddly, the children love their teddy bears.
    d. Cute and cuddly, the teddy bears are loved by many children.

33. Which of the following uses correct spelling?
    a. Jed was disatisfied with the acommodations at his hotel, so he requested another room.
    b. Jed was dissatisfied with the accommodations at his hotel, so he requested another room.
    c. Jed was dissatisfied with the accomodations at his hotel, so he requested another room.
    d. Jed was disatisfied with the accommodations at his hotel, so he requested another room.

34. Which of the following is an imperative sentence?
   a. Pennsylvania's state flag includes two draft horses and an eagle.
   b. Go down to the basement and check the hot water heater for signs of a leak.
   c. You must be so excited to have a new baby on the way!
   d. How many countries speak Spanish?

35. Which example shows correct comma usage for dates?
   a. The due date for the final paper in the course is Monday, May 16, 2016.
   b. The due date for the final paper in the course is Monday, May 16 2016.
   c. The due date for the final project in the course is Monday, May, 16, 2016.
   d. The due date for the final project in the course is Monday May 16, 2016.

36. Which sentence shows grammatically correct parallelism?
   a. The puppies enjoy chewing and to play tug-o-war.
   b. The puppies enjoy to chew and playing tug-o-war.
   c. The puppies enjoy to chew and to play tug-o-war.
   d. The puppies enjoy chewing and playing tug-o-war.

37. At last night's company function, in honor of Mr. Robertson's retirement, several employees spoke kindly about his career achievements.

In the preceding sentence, what part of speech is the word *function*?
   a. Adjective
   b. Adverb
   c. Verb
   d. Noun

38. Which of the examples uses the correct plural form?
   a. Tomatos
   b. Analysis
   c. Cacti
   d. Criterion

39. Which of the following examples uses correct punctuation?
   a. The moderator asked the candidates, "Is each of you prepared to discuss your position on global warming?".
   b. The moderator asked the candidates, "Is each of you prepared to discuss your position on global warming?"
   c. The moderator asked the candidates, 'Is each of you prepared to discuss your position on global warming?'
   d. The moderator asked the candidates, "Is each of you prepared to discuss your position on global warming"?

40. Based on the words *transfer, transact, translation, transport*, what is the meaning of the prefix *trans*?
   a. Separation
   b. All, everywhere
   c. Forward
   d. Across, beyond, over

41. In which of the following sentences does the word *part* function as an adjective?
    a. The part Brian was asked to play required many hours of research.
    b. She parts ways with the woodsman at the end of the book.
    c. The entire team played a part in the success of the project.
    d. Ronaldo is part Irish on his mother's side of the family.

42. All of Shannon's family and friends helped her to celebrate her 50th birthday at Café Sorrento. Which of the following is the complete subject of the preceding sentence?
    a. Family and friends
    b. All
    c. All of Shannon's family and friends
    d. Shannon's family and friends

43. Which of the following sentences uses second person point of view?
    a. I don't want to make plans for the weekend before I see my work schedule.
    b. She had to miss the last three yoga classes due to illness.
    c. Pluto is no longer considered a planet because it is not gravitationally dominant.
    d. Be sure to turn off all of the lights before locking up for the night.

44. As the tour group approached the bottom of Chichen Itza, the prodigious Mayan pyramid, they became nervous about climbing its distant peak.

Based on the context of the sentence, which of the following words shows the correct meaning of the word *prodigious*?
    a. Very large
    b. Famous
    c. Very old
    d. Fancy

45. Which of the following sentences correctly uses a hyphen?
    a. Last-year, many of the players felt unsure of the coach's methods.
    b. Some of the furniture she selected seemed a bit over - the - top for the space.
    c. Henry is a beagle-mix and is ready for adoption this weekend.
    d. Geena works to maintain a good relationship with her ex-husband to the benefit of their children.

46. Which of the following examples correctly uses quotation marks?
    a. "A Wrinkle in Time" was one of my favorite novels as a child.
    b. Though he is famous for his roles in films like "The Great Gatsby" and "Titanic," Leonardo DiCaprio has never won an Oscar.
    c. Sylvia Plath's poem, "Daddy" will be the subject of this week's group discussion.
    d. "The New York Times" reported that many fans are disappointed in some of the trades made by the Yankees this off-season.

47. Which of the following sentences shows correct word usage?
    a. It's often been said that work is better then rest.
    b. Its often been said that work is better then rest.
    c. It's often been said that work is better than rest.
    d. Its often been said that work is better than rest.

Directions for questions 48-49: Rewrite the sentence in your head following the directions given below. Keep in mind that your new sentence should be well written and should have essentially the same meaning as the original sentence.

48. There are many risks in firefighting, including smoke inhalation, exposure to hazardous materials, and oxygen deprivation, so firefighters are outfitted with many items that could save their lives, including a self-contained breathing apparatus.

Rewrite, beginning with <u>so, firefighters.</u>

The next words will be which of the following?
     a. are exposed to lots of dangerous situations.
     b. need to be very careful on the job.
     c. wear life-saving protective gear.
     d. have very risky jobs.

49. Though social media sites like Facebook, Instagram, and Snapchat have become increasingly popular, experts warn that teen users are exposing themselves to many dangers such as cyberbullying and predators.

Rewrite, beginning with <u>experts warn that.</u>

The next words will be which of the following?
     a. Facebook is dangerous.
     b. they are growing in popularity.
     c. teens are using them too much.
     d. they can be dangerous for teens.

50. While studying vocabulary, a student notices that the words *circumference*, *circumnavigate*, and *circumstance* all begin with the prefix *circum–*. The student uses her knowledge of affixes to infer that all of these words share what related meaning?
     a. Around, surrounding
     b. Travel, transport
     c. Size, measurement
     d. Area, location

Biology

1. Which of the following structures is unique to eukaryotic cells?
     a. Cell walls
     b. Nucleuses
     c. Cell membranes
     d. Vacuoles

2. Which is the cellular organelle used to tag, package, and ship out proteins destined for other cells or locations?
     a. The Golgi apparatus
     b. The lysosome
     c. The centrioles
     d. The mitochondria

3. Which of the following represents a helpful inherited adaptation?
    a. A male elephant defending his territory by chasing another elephant away.
    b. A female dog that has a permanent strong odor that other male dogs tend to avoid.
    c. A male moose born with bigger horns that enable him to reduce competition for mating.
    d. A monkey learning to peel a banana after several tries.

4. Esther is left-handed. Hand dominance is a genetic factor. If being right-handed is a dominant trait over being left-handed, which of the following cannot be true about Esther's parents?
    a. Her parents are both right-handed.
    b. Her parents are both left-handed.
    c. Only one parent is right-handed.
    d. All of the above can be true.

5. Cell -> ___1___ -> ___2___ -> organ system -> organism
Fill in blank #2 with the correct structure and a possible example in the circulatory system.
    a. Organ: heart
    b. Organ: blood vessel
    c. Tissue: heart
    d. Tissue: blood vessel

Use the following image to answer question 10.

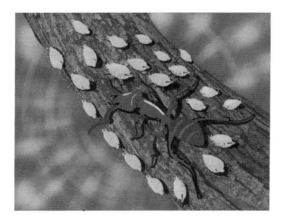

6. Ants and aphids are organisms commonly found in nature. The ant doesn't eat the aphid, nor does the aphid eat the ant, so they have a different type of relationship than predator-prey. When aphids feed on plants, they simultaneously secrete a sugary substance that ants like to snack on. Ants in return protect the aphids from predators. What kind of relationship do the ant and the aphid demonstrate?
    a. Competition
    b. Parasitism
    c. Mutualism
    d. Commensalism

7. Which definition describes an ecosystem?
    a. One individual organism
    b. Rocks, soil, and atmosphere within an area
    c. All the organisms in a food web
    d. All living and nonliving things in an area

8. What is a product of photosynthesis?
   a. Water
   b. Sunlight
   c. Oxygen
   d. Carbon Dioxide

9. What is cellular respiration?
   a. Making high-energy sugars
   b. Breathing
   c. Breaking down food to release energy
   d. Sweating

10. Which one of the following can perform photosynthesis?
    a. Mold
    b. Ant
    c. Mushroom
    d. Algae

11. What does the re-radiation of solar waves trapped in the earth's atmosphere contribute to?
    a. Global warming
    b. Greenhouse effect
    c. Climate change
    d. All of the above

Use the following image to answer questions 12 and 13.

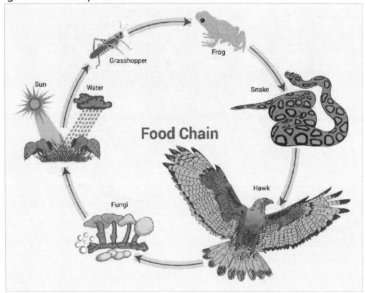

12. Which is the decomposer in the food chain above?
    a. Sun
    b. Grass
    c. Frog
    d. Fungi

13. Which is the herbivore in the food chain above?
   a. Grass
   b. Grasshopper
   c. Frog
   d. Fungi

14. When human cells divide by meiosis, how many chromosomes do the resulting cells contain?
   a. 96
   b. 54
   c. 46
   d. 23

15. Which choice is a consequence of tetrad formation in meiosis?
   a. Causes diversity
   b. Determines Gender
   c. Causes non-disjunction
   d. Causes transcription

16. Which of the following correctly expresses the molecular investment for each molecule of G3P produced by the Calvin cycle?
   a. 6 ATP molecules and 9 NADP+ molecules are invested each molecule of G3P that is produced.
   b. 9 ATP molecules and 6 NADP+ molecules are invested for each molecule of G3P that is produced.
   c. 6 ATP molecules and 9 NADPH molecules are invested for each molecule of G3P that is produced.
   d. 9 ATP molecules and 6 NADPH molecules are invested for each molecule of G3P that is produced.

17. What are the net products of anaerobic glycolysis?
   a. 2 pyruvate molecules, 2 NADH molecules, and 2 ATP molecules
   b. 2 pyruvate molecules, 2 NADH molecules, and 4 ATP molecules
   c. 2 pyruvate molecules, 2 NAD+ molecules, and 2 ATP molecules
   d. 2 pyruvate molecules, 2 NAD+ molecules, and 4 ATP molecules

18. Which of the following correctly states the relationship between the glucose molecules that initially enter into glycolysis and the number of rounds of the citric acid cycle that can be completed?
   a. One round of the citric acid cycle can be completed for each glucose molecule that enters glycolysis.
   b. One round of the citric acid cycle can be completed for every two glucose molecules that enter glycolysis.
   c. Two rounds of the citric acid cycle can be completed for each glucose molecule that enters glycolysis.
   d. One round of the citric acid cycle can be completed for every four glucose molecule that enter glycolysis.

19. What are the two steps of oxidative phosphorylation?
   a. Electron Transport Chain and Citric Acid Cycle
   b. Krebs Cycle and Electron Transport Chain
   c. Proton Pump and Facilitated Diffusion
   d. Electron Transport Chain and Chemiosmosis

20. Which of the following can be considered an animal cell analog of the plasmodesmata in terms of function?
    a. Proteoglycans
    b. Tight junction
    c. Gap junction
    d. Phospholipid bilayer

21. In which organelle do eukaryotes carry out aerobic respiration?
    a. Golgi apparatus
    b. Nucleus
    c. Mitochondrion
    d. Cytosol

22. What kind of energy do plants use in photosynthesis to create chemical energy?
    a. Light
    b. Electric
    c. Nuclear
    d. Cellular

23. What type of biological molecule is a monosaccharide?
    a. Protein
    b. Carbohydrate
    c. Nucleic acid
    d. Lipid

24. Which level of protein structure is defined by the folds and coils of the protein's polypeptide backbone?
    a. Primary
    b. Secondary
    c. Tertiary
    d. Quaternary

25. Which of the following is a representation of a natural pattern or occurrence that's difficult or impossible to experience directly?
    a. A theory
    b. A model
    c. A law
    d. An observation

Chemistry

1. How many centimeters is 0.78 kilometers?
    a. 7.8 cm
    b. 0.078 cm
    c. 78,000 cm
    d. 780 cm

2. 4.67 miles is equivalent to how many kilometers to three significant digits?
   a. 7.514 km
   b. 7.51 km
   c. 2.90 km
   d. 2.902 km

3. Which of the following must have an equal mass number?
   I. Isotopes
   II. Isotones
   III. Isobars
   a. I only
   b. I and II only
   c. II and III only
   d. III only

4. The number 0.00067 has how many significant figures?
   a. Six
   b. Five
   c. Three
   d. Two

5. The acceleration of a falling object due to gravity has been proven to be 9.8 m/s². A scientist drops a cactus four times and measures the acceleration with an accelerometer and gets the following results: 9.79 m/s², 9.81 m/s², 9.80 m/s², and 9.78 m/s². Which of the following accurately describes the measurements?
   a. They're both accurate and precise.
   b. They're accurate but not precise.
   c. They're precise but not accurate.
   d. They're neither accurate nor precise.

6. Which is the correct value for the mean of the following numbers to the appropriate number of significant figures: 3.2, 7.5, 9.6, and 5.4?
   a. 6.4
   b. 6.42
   c. 6.425
   d. 6

7. How many mL (to the appropriate number of significant figures) of a 12.0 M stock solution of HCl should be added to water to create 250 mL of a 1.50 M solution of HCl?
   a. 31.25 mL
   b. 32 mL
   c. 30 mL
   d. 31.3 mL

8. If a reading is above the curve on a solubility curve, the solvent is considered to be which of the following?
   a. Unsaturated
   b. Supersaturated
   c. Stable
   d. Saturated

9. Which of the following correctly lists the maximum number of electrons that the first three orbitals can accommodate?
   a. 2, 4, 8
   b. 1, 4. 8
   c. 2, 2, 8
   d. 2, 8, 8

10. Which of the following is true regarding Ionic bonds?
   a. The metallic substance usually transfers an electron to the nonmetal.
   b. The metallic substance often has a high electron affinity.
   c. The ionic substances formed have low melting and boiling points because of the relatively weak bonds.
   d. The formation of ionic bonds is an endothermic reaction.

11. What is the most electronegative element?
   a. Hydrogen
   b. Fluorine
   c. Oxygen
   d. Chlorine

12. In covalent bonding, how does the number of electrons involved in bonding affect bond length?
   a. The more electrons shared, the longer the bond.
   b. The more electrons shared, the shorter the bond.
   c. The more electrons transferred, the longer the bond.
   d. The more electrons transferred, the shorter the bond.

13. Which is the term for a homogeneous mixture that does not have the Tyndall effect?
   a. Solvent
   b. Suspension
   c. Solution
   d. Colloid

14. Which of the following statements is true regarding Lewis structures for metallic compounds?
   a. Lewis structures are most accurate for metallic compounds because of the natural way electrons in metallic substances arrange themselves in rather predictable, geometric arrangements.
   b. Lewis structures are not common for metallic compounds because of the free-roaming ability of the electrons.
   c. A Lewis symbol for an element entering a metallic bond can have dots on just the bonded side of the compound, for a maximum of two dots.
   d. Lewis structures help visualize the electrons in metallic compounds more easily than in covalent structures, where the electron sharing cannot be depicted well.

15. What is ionization energy?
    a. One-half the distance between the nuclei of atoms of the same element.
    b. A measurement of the willingness of an atom to form a chemical bond.
    c. The amount of energy needed to remove a valence electron from a gas or ion.
    d. The ability or tendency of an atom to accept an electron into its valence shell.

16. For gaseous reactants, how does decreasing the pressure in the system affect the reaction rate?
    a. The reaction rate increases because the frequency of collisions increases.
    b. The reaction rate increases because the frequency of collisions decreases.
    c. The reaction rate decreases because the frequency of collisions increases.
    d. The reaction rate decreases because the frequency of collisions decreases.

17. What can be said about the reaction described by the following generic chemical equation?

$$aA \text{ (s)} + bB \text{ (aq)} \leftrightarrow cC \text{ (s)} + dD \text{ (aq)}$$

    a. The reaction is in static equilibrium.
    b. The reaction is in dynamic equilibrium.
    c. The reaction is in heterogenous equilibrium.
    d. The reaction is in homogenous equilibrium.

18. Based on collision theory, what is the effect of temperature on the rate of chemical reaction?
    a. Increasing the temperature slows the reaction.
    b. Decreasing the temperature speeds up the reaction.
    c. Increasing the temperature speeds up the reaction.
    d. Collision theory and temperature are unrelated.

19. Burning a piece of paper is what type of change?
    a. Chemical change
    b. Physical change
    c. Sedimentary change
    d. Potential change

20. Which of the following is true?
    a. A base acts as a proton donor in a chemical equation.
    b. A base is an electron-pair acceptor in a chemical equation.
    c. An acid increases the concentration of H^+ ions when it is dissolved in water.
    d. An acid increases the concentration of OH^- ions when it is dissolved in water.

21. Which of the following is a synthesis reaction?
    a. $2NO + O_2 \rightarrow 2NO_2$
    b. $H_2CO_3 \rightarrow H_2O + CO_2$
    c. $Mg + 2HCl \rightarrow MgCl_2 + H_2$
    d. $Zn + 2 HCl \rightarrow ZnCl_2 + H_2$

22. What type of reaction is $CH_4 + 2O_2 \rightarrow CO_2 + 2H_2O$?
    a. Substitution Reaction
    b. Combustion Reaction
    c. Redox Reaction
    d. Acid-Base Reaction

23. What is the percent yield for the reaction that produces 45 grams of CaO if 65 grams were expected out of the reaction $CaCO_3 \rightarrow CaO + CO_2$?

    a. 6.9%

    b. 69%

    c. 144%

    d. 14.4%

24. Which of the following statements is true?

    a. When an atom, ion, or molecule loses its electrons and becomes more positively charged, it has been reduced.

    b. When an atom, ion, or molecule loses its electrons and becomes more positively charged, it has been oxidized.

    c. When an atom, ion, or molecule loses its electrons and becomes more negatively charged, it has been oxidized.

    d. When an atom, ion, or molecule loses its electrons and becomes more negatively charged, it has been reduced.

25. Which of the following correctly shows a conjugate acid paired with its conjugate base?

    a. H_2SO_4 (acid) and HSO_4^- (conjugate base)

    b. HSO_4^- (acid) and H_2SO_4 (conjugate base)

    c. H_2SO_4 (acid) and HSO_4^+ (conjugate base)

    d. HSO_4^+ (acid) and H_2SO_4 (conjugate base)

Anatomy and Physiology

1. Retinacular connective tissue serves what primary purpose?

    a. Support

    b. Flexibility

    c. Strength

    d. Lubrication

2. Which of the following is one of the functions of the stratum basale layer of the epidermis?

    a. Repelling water

    b. Protecting against UV rays

    c. Producing keratin

    d. Producing oil to lubricate and protect the skin

3. Why do arteries have valves?

    a. They have valves to maintain high blood pressure so that capillaries diffuse nutrients properly.

    b. Their valves are designed to prevent backflow due to their low blood pressure.

    c. They have valves due to a leftover trait from evolution that, like the appendix, are useless.

    d. They do not have valves, but veins do.

4. How does cartilage obtain nutrients?

    a. A network of fine capillaries

    b. An extensive network of internal vasculature

    c. Carrier proteins

    d. Diffusion

5. In terms of levels of organization in the body, the next level up from cells is which of the following? In other words, groups of cells are arranged into which of the following?
   a. Organ systems
   b. Atoms
   c. Organs
   d. Tissues

6. Which of the following is NOT one of the functions of sebum?
   a. Protecting the skin from water loss
   b. Moisturizing the skin
   c. Helping with thermoregulation by assisting with evaporative cooling
   d. Providing a chemical defense against bacterial and fungal infections

7. Which of the following statements accurately describes the basics of the sliding filament model of muscle contraction?
   a. Myosin filaments form and break cross-bridges with actin in order to pull the actin filaments closer to the M line.
   b. Actin filaments form and break cross-bridges with myosin in order to pull the myosin filaments closer to the M line.
   c. Myosin filaments form and break cross-bridges with actin in order to pull the actin filaments closer to the Z line.
   d. Actin filaments form and break cross-bridges with myosin in order to pull the myosin filaments closer to the Z line.

8. What is one of the characteristics of transitional epithelial tissue that differentiates it from other types of epithelial tissue?
   a. It is composed solely from a single layer of cells.
   b. It appears to be stratified but actually consists of only one layer of cells.
   c. It helps protect the body from invasions of microbes like bacteria and parasites.
   d. It can expand and contract.

9. What structures are made by the body's white blood cells that fight bacterial infections?
   a. Antibodies
   b. Antibiotics
   c. Vaccines
   d. Red blood cells

10. Which blood component is chiefly responsible for oxygen transport?
    a. Platelets
    b. Red blood cells
    c. White blood cells
    d. Plasma cells

11. Which is the first event to happen in a primary immune response?
    a. Macrophages phagocytose pathogens and present their antigens.
    b. Neutrophils aggregate and act as cytotoxic, nonspecific killers of pathogens.
    c. B lymphocytes make pathogen-specific antibodies.
    d. Helper T cells secrete interleukins to activate pathogen-fighting cells.

12. Where does sperm maturation take place in the male reproductive system?
    a. Seminal vesicles
    b. Prostate gland
    c. Epididymis
    d. Vas Deferens

13. Which hormone in the female reproductive system is responsible for progesterone production?
    a. FSH
    b. LH
    c. hCG
    d. Estrogen

14. Which epithelial tissue comprises the cell layer found in a capillary bed?
    a. Squamous
    b. Cuboidal
    c. Columnar
    d. Stratified

15. When considering anatomical direction, what is the position of the clavicle to the humerus?
    a. Lateral
    b. Medial
    c. Distal
    d. Inferior

16. What is the body plane that runs vertically through the body at right angles to the midline?
    a. Coronal
    b. Transverse
    c. Sagittal
    d. Superior

17. Which statement is true?
    a. Ligaments attach skeletal muscles to bone.
    b. Tendons connect bones at joints.
    c. Cartilage adds mechanical support to joints.
    d. Most veins deliver oxygenated blood to cells.

18. Which layer of skin contains sensory receptors and blood vessels?
    a. Epidermis
    b. Dermis
    c. Hypodermis
    d. Subcutaneous

19. Receptors in the dermis help the body maintain homeostasis by relaying messages to what area of the brain?
    a. The cerebellum
    b. The brain stem
    c. The pituitary gland
    d. The hypothalamus

20. The radius and ulna are to the humerus what the tibia and fibula are to the _____.
    a. Mandible
    b. Femur
    c. Scapula
    d. Carpal

21. What are concentric circles of bone tissue are called?
    a. Lacunae
    b. Lamellae
    c. Trabeculae
    d. Diaphysis

22. When de-oxygenated blood first enters the heart, which of the following choices is in the correct order for its journey to the aorta?
    I. Tricuspid valve → Lungs → Mitral valve
    II. Mitral valve → Lungs → Tricuspid valve
    III. Right ventricle → Lungs → Left atrium
    IV. Left ventricle → Lungs → Right atrium
    a. I and III only
    b. I and IV only
    c. II and III only
    d. II and IV only

23. Which characteristics are true for skeletal muscle?
    I. Contain sarcomeres
    II. Have multiple nuclei
    III. Are branched
    a. I only
    b. I and II only
    c. I, II, and III only
    d. II and III only

24. Which is the simplest nerve pathway that bypasses the brain?
    a. Autonomic
    b. Reflex arc
    c. Somatic
    d. Sympathetic

25. What makes bone resistant to shattering?
    a. The calcium salts deposited in the bone
    b. The collagen fibers
    c. The bone marrow and network of blood vessels
    d. The intricate balance of minerals and collagen fibers

Physics

1. The heat transfer due to the movement of gas molecules from an area of higher concentration to one of lower concentration is known as what?
    a. Conduction
    b. Convection
    c. Solarization
    d. Radiation

2. Which of the following is true of an object at rest on Earth?
    a. It has no forces acting upon it.
    b. It has no gravity acting upon it.
    c. It is in transition.
    d. It is in equilibrium.

3. What is a change in state from a solid to a gas called?
    a. Evaporation
    b. Melting
    c. Condensation
    d. Sublimation

4. Which is not a form of energy?
    a. Light
    b. Sound
    c. Heat
    d. Mass

5. A projectile at a point along its path has 30 Joules of potential energy and 20 Joules of kinetic energy. What is the total mechanical energy for the projectile?
    a. 50 Joules
    b. 30 Joules
    c. 20 Joules
    d. 10 Joules

6. Why would a pencil appear to bend at the water line in a glass of water?
    a. The wood of the pencil becomes warped from being in the water.
    b. It appears to bend because of the refraction of light traveling from air to water.
    c. The pencil temporarily bends because of its immersion into separate mediums.
    d. The reflection of the light from water to a human's pupil creates the illusion of a warping object.

7. What is the current when a 3.0 V battery is wired across a lightbulb that has a resistance of 6.0 ohms?
    a. 0.5 A
    b. 18.0 A
    c. 0.5 J
    d. 18.0 J

8. The law of the conservation of energy states which of the following?
    a. Energy should be stored in power cells for future use.
    b. Energy will replenish itself once exhausted.
    c. Energy cannot be created or destroyed.
    d. Energy should be saved because it can run out.

9. Running electricity through a wire generates which of the following?
    a. A gravitational field
    b. A frictional field
    c. An acoustic field
    d. A magnetic field

10. What is the total mechanical energy of a system?
    a. The total potential energy
    b. The total kinetic energy
    c. Kinetic energy plus potential energy
    d. Kinetic energy minus potential energy

Answer Explanations

Mathematics

1. D: $\frac{3}{100}$. Each digit to the left of the decimal point represents a higher multiple of 10 and each digit to the right of the decimal point represents a quotient of a higher multiple of 10 for the divisor. The first digit to the right of the decimal point is equal to the value ÷ 10. The second digit to the right of the decimal point is equal to the value ÷ (10 × 10), or the value ÷ 100.

2. B: 102,317

Set up the problem and add each column, starting on the far right (ones). Add, carrying anything over 9 into the next column to the left. Solve from right to left.

3. A: 847.90. The hundredth place value is located two digits to the right of the decimal point (the digit 9). The digit to the right of the place value is examined to decide whether to round up or keep the digit. In this case, the digit 6 is 5 or greater so the hundredth place is rounded up. When rounding up, if the digit to be increased is a 9, the digit to its left is increased by one and the digit in the desired place value is made a zero. Therefore, the number is rounded to 847.90.

4. B: $\frac{11}{15}$. Fractions must have like denominators to be added. The least common multiple of the denominators 3 and 5 is found. The LCM is 15, so both fractions should be changed to equivalent fractions with a denominator of 15. To determine the numerator of the new fraction, the old numerator is multiplied by the same number by which the old denominator is multiplied to obtain the new denominator. For the fraction $\frac{1}{3}$, 3 multiplied by 5 will produce 15. Therefore, the numerator is multiplied by 5 to produce the new numerator $\left(\frac{1\times5}{3\times5} = \frac{5}{15}\right)$. For the fraction $\frac{2}{5}$, multiplying both the numerator and denominator by 3 produces $\frac{6}{15}$. When fractions have like denominators, they are added by adding the numerators and keeping the denominator the same: $\frac{5}{15} + \frac{6}{15} = \frac{11}{15}$.

5. A: $1\frac{5}{36}$

Set up the problem and find a common denominator for both fractions.

$$\frac{7}{12} + \frac{5}{9}$$

Multiply each fraction to convert to a common denominator.

$$\frac{7}{12} \times \frac{3}{3} + \frac{5}{9} \times \frac{4}{4}$$

Once over the same denominator, add across the top. The total is over the common denominator.

$$\frac{21 + 20}{36} = \frac{41}{36}$$

Convert to a mixed number.

$$\frac{41}{36} = 1\frac{5}{36}$$

6. D: 80%. To convert a fraction to a percent, the fraction is first converted to a decimal. To do so, the numerator is divided by the denominator: $4 \div 5 = 0.8$. To convert a decimal to a percent, the number is multiplied by 100: $0.8 \times 100 = 80\%$.

7. D: 6,258

Set up the problem, with the larger number on top. Begin subtracting with the far right column (ones). Borrow 10 from the column to the left when necessary.

8. D: 1, 2, 3, 4, 6, 12. A given number divides evenly by each of its factors to produce an integer (no decimals). The number 5, 7, 8, 9, 10, 11 (and their opposites) do not divide evenly into 12. Therefore, these numbers are not factors.

9. A: 11. To determine the number of houses that can fit on the street, the length of the street is divided by the width of each house: $345 \div 30 = 11.5$. Although the mathematical calculation of 11.5 is correct, this answer is not reasonable. Half of a house cannot be built, so the company will need to either build 11 or 12 houses. Since the width of 12 houses (360 feet) will extend past the length of the street, only 11 houses can be built.

10. C: 594.02

Set up the problem, with the larger number on top and numbers lined up at the decimal. Insert 0 in any blank spots to the right of the decimal as placeholders. Begin subtracting with the far right column. Borrow 10 from the column to the left when necessary.

11. A: $\frac{5}{8}$

Set up the problem and find a common denominator for both fractions.

$$\frac{19}{24} - \frac{1}{6}$$

Multiply the second fraction to convert to a common denominator.

$$\frac{19}{24} - \frac{1}{6} \times \frac{4}{4}$$

Once over the same denominator, subtract across the top.

$$\frac{19 - 4}{24} = \frac{15}{24}$$

Reduce by dividing the numerator and denominator by a common factor (3).

$$\frac{15}{24} = \frac{5}{8}$$

12. D: $x \leq -5$. When solving a linear equation or inequality:

Distribution is performed if necessary: $-3(x + 4) \rightarrow -3x - 12 \geq x + 8$. This means that any like terms on the same side of the equation/inequality are combined.

The equation/inequality is manipulated to get the variable on one side. In this case, subtracting x from both sides produces $-4x - 12 \geq 8$.

The variable is isolated using inverse operations to undo addition/subtraction. Adding 12 to both sides produces $-4x \geq 20$.

The variable is isolated using inverse operations to undo multiplication/division. Remember if dividing by a negative number, the relationship of the inequality reverses, so the sign is flipped. In this case, dividing by -4 on both sides produces $x \leq -5$.

13. C: 4,498

Line up the numbers (the number with the most digits on top) to multiply. Begin with the left column on top and the left column on bottom.

Move one column left on top and multiply by the far right column on the bottom. Remember to carry over after you multiply.

Starting on the far right column, on top, repeat this pattern for the next number left on the bottom. Write the answers below the first line of answers. Remember to begin with a zero placeholder.

Continue the pattern.

Add the answer rows together, making sure they are still lined up correctly.

14. D: $x > 2$. The open dot on one indicates that the value is not included in the set. The arrow pointing right indicates that numbers greater than two (numbers get larger to the right) are included in the set. Therefore, the set includes numbers greater than two, which can be written as $x > 2$.

15. A: o. The core of the pattern consists of 4 items: ▲oo□. Therefore, the core repeats in multiples of 4, with the pattern starting over on the next step. The closest multiple of 4 to 42 is 40. Step 40 is the end of the core (□), so step 41 will start the core over (▲) and step 42 is o.

16. B: Instead of multiplying these out, the product can be estimated by using $18 \times 10 = 180$. The error here should be lower than 15, since it is rounded to the nearest integer, and the numbers add to something less than 30.

17. D: 40% is $\frac{4}{10}$. The number itself must be $\frac{10}{4}$ of 12, or $\frac{10}{4} \times 12 = 10 \times 3 = 30$.

18. A: Convert these numbers to improper fractions: $\frac{11}{3} - \frac{9}{5}$. Take 15 as a common denominator: $\frac{11}{3} - \frac{9}{5} = \frac{55}{15} - \frac{27}{15} = \frac{28}{15} = 1\frac{13}{15}$ (when rewritten to get rid of the partial fraction).

19. C: Dividing by 100 means shifting the decimal point of the numerator to the left by 2. The result is 6.6 and rounds to 7.

20. B: Because these decimals are all negative, the number that is the largest will be the number whose absolute value is the smallest, as that will be the negative number with the least value. Thus, it will be the "least negative" (closest to zero). To figure out which number has the smallest absolute value, look at the first non-zero digits. The first nonzero digit in Choice *B* is in the hundredths place. The other three all have nonzero digits in the tenths place, so Choice *B* is closest to zero; thus, it is the largest of the four negative numbers.

21. C: To solve for the value of b, both sides of the equation need to be equalized.

Start by cancelling out the lower value of -4 by adding 4 to both sides:

$$5b - 4 = 2b + 17$$
$$5b - 4 + 4 = 2b + 17 + 4$$
$$5b = 2b + 21$$

The variable *b* is the same on each side, so subtract the lower 2b from each side:

$$5b = 2b + 21$$
$$5b - 2b = 2b + 21 - 2b$$
$$3b = 21$$

Then divide both sides by 3 to get the value of *b*:

$$3b = 21$$

$$\frac{3b}{3} = \frac{21}{3}$$

$$b = 7$$

22. C: $\frac{1}{3}$ of the shirts sold were patterned. Therefore, $1 - \frac{1}{3} = \frac{2}{3}$ of the shirts sold were solid. Anytime "of" a quantity appears in a word problem, multiplication should be used.

Therefore:

$$192 \times \frac{2}{3} = \frac{192 \times 2}{3} = \frac{384}{3} = 128 \text{ solid shirts were sold}$$

The entire expression is $192 \times \left(1 - \frac{1}{3}\right)$.

23. A: Mean. An outlier is a data value that is either far above or far below the majority of values in a sample set. The mean is the average of all the values in the set. In a small sample set, a very high or very low number could drastically change the average of the data points. Outliers will have no more of an effect on the median (the middle value when arranged from lowest to highest) than any other value above or below the median. If the same outlier does not repeat, outliers will have no effect on the mode (value that repeats most often).

24. A: 13/5

Set up the division problem.

$$\frac{5}{13} \div \frac{25}{169}$$

Flip the second fraction and multiply.

$$\frac{5}{13} \times \frac{169}{25}$$

Simplify and reduce with cross multiplication.

$$\frac{1}{1} \times \frac{13}{5}$$

Multiply across the top and across the bottom to solve.

$$\frac{1 \times 13}{1 \times 5} = \frac{13}{5}$$

25. A: 3 3/5

Divide.

$$15\overline{)54}$$
$$\underline{-45}$$
$$9$$

The result is 3 9/15.

Reduce the remainder for the final answer.

3 3/5

26. A: Using the order of operations, multiplication and division are computed first from left to right. Multiplication is on the left; therefore, the teacher should perform multiplication first.

27. D: 59/7

The original number was 8 3/7. Multiply the denominator by the whole number portion. Add the numerator and put the total over the original denominator.

$$\frac{(8 \times 7) + 3}{7} = \frac{59}{7}$$

28. B: 93/8

The original number was 11 5/8. Multiply the denominator by the whole number portion. Add the numerator and put the total over the original denominator.

$$\frac{(8 \times 11) + 5}{8} = \frac{93}{8}$$

29. B: 8.1

To round 8.067 to the nearest tenths, use the digit in the hundredths.

6 in the hundredths is greater than 5, so round up in the tenths.

8.0<u>6</u>7

0 becomes a 1.

8.1

30. A: The place value to the right of the thousandth place, which would be the ten-thousandth place, is what gets used. The value in the thousandth place is 7. The number in the place value to its right is greater than 4, so the 7 gets bumped up to 8. Everything to its right turns to a zero, to get 245.2680. The zero is dropped because it is part of the decimal.

31. B: This is a division problem because the original amount needs to be split up into equal amounts. The mixed number $12\frac{1}{2}$ should be converted to an improper fraction first. $12\frac{1}{2} = \frac{(12*2)+1}{2} = \frac{23}{2}$. Carey needs determine how many times $\frac{23}{2}$ goes into 184. This is a division problem: $184 \div \frac{23}{2} =?$ The fraction can be flipped, and the problem turns into the multiplication: $184 \times \frac{2}{23} = \frac{368}{23}$. This improper fraction can be simplified into 16 because $368 \div 23 = 16$. The answer is 16 lawn segments.

32. B: 100 cm is equal to 1 m. 1.3 divided by 100 is 0.013. Therefore, 1.3 cm is equal to 0.013 mm. Because 1 cm is equal to 10 mm, 1.3 cm is equal to 13 mm.

33. B: Using the conversion rate, the projected weight loss of 25 pounds is multiplied by 0.45 $\frac{kg}{lb}$ to get the amount in kilograms (11.25 kg).

34. D: Start by taking a common denominator of 30. $\frac{14}{15} = \frac{28}{30}, \frac{3}{5} = \frac{18}{30}, \frac{1}{30} = \frac{1}{30}$. Add and subtract the numerators for the next step. $\frac{28}{30} + \frac{18}{30} - \frac{1}{30} = \frac{28+18-1}{30} = \frac{45}{30} = \frac{3}{2}$, where in the last step the 15 is factored out from the numerator and denominator.

35. C: First, the square root of 16 is 4. So this simplifies to $\frac{1}{2}\sqrt{16} = \frac{1}{2}(4) = 2$.

36. C: DXVII

Break down the number into parts.

517 = 500 + 10 + 5 + 2

500 is represented by D or 500 = D

10 is represented by X or 10 = X

5 is represented by V or 5 = V

2 is represented by II.

Combine the Roman numerals.

DXVii

37. A: 3:00 p.m.

Since military time starts with 0100 at 1:00 a.m., add 14 to get to 1500 hours, or 3:00 p.m.

38. D: To take the product of two fractions, just multiply the numerators and denominators. $\frac{5}{3} \times \frac{7}{6} = \frac{5 \times 7}{3 \times 6} = \frac{35}{18}$. The numerator and denominator have no common factors, so this is simplified completely.

39. A: A common denominator must be found. The least common denominator is 15 because it has both 5 and 3 as factors. The fractions must be rewritten using 15 as the denominator.

40. B: 1000 hours

Anything before noon converts over from its a.m. value.

41. D: 100,000.0 cm

To convert from kilometers to centimeters, move the decimal 5 places to the right.

1.0 Km = 100000.0 cm

42. A: Operations within the parentheses must be completed first. Then, division is completed. Finally, addition is the last operation to complete. When adding decimals, digits within each place value are added together. Therefore, the expression is evaluated as $(2 \times 20) \div (7 + 1) + (6 \times 0.01) + (4 \times 0.001) = 40 \div 8 + 0.06 + 0.004 = 5 + 0.06 + 0.004 = 5.064$.

43. B: $-\frac{1}{3}\sqrt{81} = -\frac{1}{3}(9) = -3$

44. C: A dollar contains 20 nickels. Therefore, if there are 12 dollars' worth of nickels, there are $12 \times 20 = 240$ nickels. Each nickel weighs 5 grams. Therefore, the weight of the nickels is $240 \times 5 = 1,200$ grams. Adding in the weight of the empty piggy bank, the filled bank weighs 2,250 grams.

45. D: 3 must be multiplied times $27\frac{3}{4}$. In order to easily do this, the mixed number should be converted into an improper fraction. $27\frac{3}{4} = \frac{27*4+3}{4} = \frac{111}{4}$. Therefore, Denver had approximately $\frac{3x111}{4} = \frac{333}{4}$ inches of snow. The improper fraction can be converted back into a mixed number through division. $\frac{333}{4} = 83\frac{1}{4}$ inches.

46. C: 120 pts

List out and set up equivalencies.

$$8 \, pts. = 1 \, gal.$$

Set up the equivalencies with the initial values.

$$\frac{15 \, gal}{1} \times \frac{8 \, pts}{1 \, gal}$$

Cross-cancel units then multiply across the top and the bottom.

$$\frac{15 \times 8 \, pts}{1} = 120 \, pts$$

47. B: 99. 32 °F

Set up the equation for converting Celsius to Fahrenheit.

$$F = (9/5)\,C + 32$$

Fill in the givens.

$$F = (9/5)\,37.4 + 32$$

Solve the equation in in parentheses. Multiply, then add.

$$F = 67.32 + 32$$

$$F = 99.32\ ^0F$$

48. D: To find the average of a set of values, the values are added together and then this sum is divided by the total number of values. In this case, the unknown value of what Dwayne needs to score on his next test needs to be added, in order to solve it.

$$\frac{78 + 92 + 83 + 97 + x}{5} = 90$$

The unknown value is added to the new average total, which is 5. Then, each side is multiplied by 5 to simplify the equation, resulting in:

$$78 + 92 + 83 + 97 + x = 450$$

$$350 + x = 450$$

$$x = 100$$

Dwayne would need to get a perfect score of 100 in order to get an average of at least 90.

This answer can be confirmed by substituting it back into the original formula.

$$\frac{78 + 92 + 83 + 97 + 100}{5} = 90$$

49. C: For an even number of total values, the *median* is calculated by finding the *mean* or average of the two middle values once all values have been arranged in ascending order from least to greatest. In this case, $(92 + 83) \div 2$ would equal the median 87.5, Choice C.

50. D: The expression is three times the sum of twice a number and 1, which is $3(2x + 1)$. Then, 6 is subtracted from this expression.

Reading Comprehension

1. C: Gulliver becomes acquainted with the people and practices of his new surroundings. Choice C is the correct answer because it most extensively summarizes the entire passage. While Choices A and B are reasonable possibilities, they reference portions of Gulliver's experiences, not the whole. Choice D is incorrect because Gulliver doesn't express repentance or sorrow in this particular passage.

2. A: Principal refers to *chief* or *primary* within the context of this text. Choice *A* is the answer that most closely aligns with this answer. Choices *B* and *D* make reference to a helper or followers while Choice *C* doesn't meet the description of Gulliver from the passage.

3. C: One can reasonably infer that Gulliver is considerably larger than the children who were playing around him because multiple children could fit into his hand. Choice *B* is incorrect because there is no indication of stress in Gulliver's tone. Choices *A* and *D* aren't the best answer because though Gulliver seems fond of his new acquaintances, he didn't travel there with the intentions of meeting new people or to express a definite love for them in this particular portion of the text.

4. C: The emperor made a *definitive decision* to expose Gulliver to their native customs. In this instance, the word *mind* was not related to a vote, question, or cognitive ability.

5. A: Choice *A* is correct. This assertion does *not* support the fact that games are a commonplace event in this culture because it mentions conduct, not games. Choices *B, C,* and *D* are incorrect because these do support the fact that games were a commonplace event.

6. B: Choice *B* is the only option that mentions the correlation between physical ability and leadership positions. Choices *A* and *D* are unrelated to physical strength and leadership abilities. Choice *C* does not make a deduction that would lead to the correct answer—it only comments upon the abilities of common townspeople.

7. D: To enlighten the audience on the habits of sun-fish and their hatcheries. Choice *A* is incorrect because although the Adirondack region is mentioned in the text, there is no cause or effect relationships between the region and fish hatcheries depicted here. Choice *B* is incorrect because the text does not have an agenda, but rather is meant to inform the audience. Finally, Choice *C* is incorrect because the text says nothing of how sun-fish mate.

8. B: The sun-fish builds it with her tail and snout. The text explains this in the second paragraph: "she builds, with her tail and snout, a circular embankment 3 inches in height and 2 thick." Choice *A* is used in the text as a simile.

9. D: To conclude a sequence and add a final detail. The concluding sequence is expressed in the phrase "[t]he mother sun-fish, having now built or provided her 'hatchery.'" The final detail is the way in which the sun-fish guards the "inclosure." Choices *A, B,* and *C* are incorrect.

10. C: *Extraneous* most nearly means *superfluous,* or *trivial.* Choice *A, indispensable,* is incorrect because it means the opposite of *extraneous.* Choice *B, bewildering,* means *confusing* and is not relevant to the context of the sentence. Finally, Choice *D* is wrong because although the prefix of the word is the same, *ex-,* the word *exuberant* means *elated* or *enthusiastic,* and is irrelevant to the context of the sentence.

11. A: Bring to light an alternative view on human perception by examining the role of technology in human understanding. This is a challenging question because the author's purpose is somewhat open-ended. The author concludes by stating that the questions regarding human perception and observation can be approached from many angles. Thus they do not seem to be attempting to prove one thing or another. Choice *B* is clearly wrong because we cannot know for certain whether the electron experiment is the latest discovery in astroparticle physics because no date is given. Choice *C* is a broad generalization that does not reflect accurately on the writer's views. While the author does appear to reflect on opposing views of human understanding (Choice *D*), the best answer is Choice *A.*

12. C: It presents a problem, explains the details of that problem, and then ends with more inquiry. The beginning of this paragraph literally "presents a conundrum," explains the problem of partial understanding, and then ends with more questions, or inquiry. There is no solution offered in this paragraph, making Choices A and B incorrect. Choice D is incorrect because the paragraph does not begin with a definition.

13. D: Looking back in the text, the author describes that classical philosophy holds that understanding can be reached by careful observation. This will not work if they are overly invested or biased in their pursuit. Choices A and C are in no way related and are completely unnecessary. A specific theory is not necessary to understanding, according to classical philosophy mentioned by the author. Again, the key to understanding is observing the phenomena outside of it, without biased or predisposition. Thus, Choice B is wrong.

14. B: The electrons passed through both holes and then onto the plate. Choices A and C are wrong because such movement is not mentioned at all in the text. In the passage the author says that electrons that were physically observed appeared to pass through one hole or another. Remember, the electrons that were observed doing this were described as acting like particles. Therefore Choice D is wrong. Recall that the plate actually recorded electrons passing through both holes simultaneously and hitting the plate. This behavior, the electron activity that wasn't seen by humans, was characteristic of waves. Thus, Choice B is the right answer.

15. D: The author explains that Boethianism is a Medieval theological philosophy that attributes sin to temporary pleasure and righteousness with virtue and God's providence. Besides Choice D, the choices listed are all physical things. While these could still be divine rewards, Boethianism holds that the true reward for being virtuous is in God's favor. It is also stressed in the article that physical pleasures cannot be taken into the afterlife. Therefore, the best choice is D, God's favor.

16. C: *The Canterbury Tales* presents a manuscript written in the medieval period that can help illustrate Boethianism through stories and show how people of the time might have responded to the idea. Choices A and B are generalized statements, and we have no evidence to support Choice B. Choice D is very compelling, but it looks at Boethianism in a way that the author does not. The author does not mention "different levels of Boethianism" when discussing the tales, only that the concept appears differently in different tales. Boethianism also doesn't focus on enlightenment.

17. D: The author is referring to the principle that a desire for material goods leads to moral malfeasance punishable by a higher being. Choice A is incorrect; while the text does mention thieves ravaging others' possessions, it is only meant as an example and not as the principle itself. Choice B is incorrect for the same reason as A. Choice C is mentioned in the text and is part of the example that proves the principle, and also not the principle itself.

18. C: The word *avarice* most nearly means *parsimoniousness*, or an unwillingness to spend money. Choice A means *evil* or *mischief* and does not relate to the context of the sentence. Choice B is also incorrect, because *pithiness* means *shortness* or *conciseness*. Choice D is close because *precariousness* means dangerous or instability, which goes well with the context. However, we are told of the summoner's specific characteristic of greed, which makes Choice C the best answer.

19. D: Desire for pleasure can lead toward sin. Boethianism acknowledges desire as something that leads out of holiness, so Choice A is incorrect. Choice B is incorrect because in the passage, Boethianism is depicted as being wary of desire and anything that binds people to the physical world. Choice C can be eliminated because the author never says that desire indicates demonic.

20. D: It emphasizes Mr. Utterson's anguish in failing to identify Hyde's whereabouts. Context clues indicate that Choice *D* is correct because the passage provides great detail of Mr. Utterson's feelings about locating Hyde. Choice *A* does not fit because there is no mention of Mr. Lanyon's mental state. Choice *B* is incorrect; although the text does make mention of bells, Choice *B* is not the *best* answer overall. Choice *C* is incorrect because the passage clearly states that Mr. Utterson was determined, not unsure.

21. A: In the city. The word *city* appears in the passage several times, thus establishing the location for the reader.

22. B: It scares children. The passage states that the Juggernaut causes the children to scream. Choices *A* and *D* don't apply because the text doesn't mention either of these instances specifically. Choice *C* is incorrect because there is nothing in the text that mentions space travel.

23. B: To constantly visit. The mention of *morning*, *noon*, and *night* make it clear that the word *haunt* refers to frequent appearances at various locations. Choice *A* doesn't work because the text makes no mention of levitating. Choices *C* and *D* are not correct because the text makes mention of Mr. Utterson's anguish and disheartenment because of his failure to find Hyde but does not make mention of Mr. Utterson's feelings negatively affecting anyone else.

24. D: This is an example of alliteration. Choice *D* is the correct answer because of the repetition of the *L*-words. Hyperbole is an exaggeration, so Choice *A* doesn't work. No comparison is being made, so no simile or metaphor is being used, thus eliminating Choices *B* and *C*.

25. D: The speaker intends to continue to look for Hyde. Choices *A* and *B* are not possible answers because the text doesn't refer to any name changes or an identity crisis, despite Mr. Utterson's extreme obsession with finding Hyde. The text also makes no mention of a mistaken identity when referring to Hyde, so Choice *C* is also incorrect.

26. D: The use of "I" could have all of the effects for the reader; it could serve to have a "hedging" effect, allow the reader to connect with the author in a more personal way, and cause the reader to empathize more with the egrets. However, it doesn't distance the reader from the text, thus eliminating Choice *D*.

27. C: The quote provides an example of a warden protecting one of the colonies. Choice *A* is incorrect because the speaker of the quote is a warden, not a hunter. Choice *B* is incorrect because the quote does not lighten the mood, but shows the danger of the situation between the wardens and the hunters. Choice *D* is incorrect because there is no humor found in the quote.

28. D: A *rookery* is a colony of breeding birds. Although *rookery* could mean Choice *A*, houses in a slum area, it does not make sense in this context. Choices *B* and *C* are both incorrect, as this is not a place for hunters to trade tools or for wardens to trade stories.

29. B: An important bird colony. The previous sentence is describing "twenty colonies" of birds, so what follows should be a bird colony. Choice *A* may be true, but we have no evidence of this in the text. Choice *C* does touch on the tension between the hunters and wardens, but there is no official "Bird Island Battle" mentioned in the text. Choice *D* does not exist in the text.

30. D: To demonstrate the success of the protective work of the Audubon Association. The text mentions several different times how and why the association has been successful and gives examples to back this fact. Choice *A* is incorrect because although the article, in some instances, calls certain people to act, it is not the purpose of the entire passage. There is no way to tell if Choices *B* and *C* are correct, as they are not mentioned in the text.

31. C: To have a better opportunity to hunt the birds. Choice *A* might be true in a general sense, but it is not relevant to the context of the text. Choice *B* is incorrect because the hunters are not studying lines of flight to help wardens, but to hunt birds. Choice *D* is incorrect because nothing in the text mentions that hunters are trying to build homes underneath lines of flight of birds for good luck.

32. D: Choice *D* correctly summarizes Frost's theme of life's journey and the choices one makes. While Choice *A* can be seen as an interpretation, it is a literal one and is incorrect. Literal is not symbolic. Choice *B* presents the idea of good and evil as a theme, and the poem does not specify this struggle for the traveler. Choice *C* is a similarly incorrect answer. Love is not the theme.

33. C: There are 20 lines in this poem. You can see the number of lines to the right of the poem (it goes to 20), or you can count the lines individually.

34. A: This poem is made up of one stanza. Lines in poems are the individual lines that break from one line to the next. Stanzas are groups of lines. If this poem had another stanza, we would see a space between a group of lines, almost like a paragraph. This poem has only one block of lines.

35. A: There is only one traveler in the poem. We see this in the line "And be one traveler, long I stood." This indicates that the speaker is alone and traveling without a partner.

36. B: The time of day in the poem is morning. The line we see this in says, "And both that morning equally lay." This question relies on how carefully the passage was read.

37. B: The traveler took the second road. We see the traveler unsure at first about whether to take the first or second road. After they choose the second road, they contemplate saving "the first for another day," but they never take the first road in the poem.

38. B: Only Choice *B* uses both repetitive beginning sounds (alliteration) and personification—the portrayal of a building as a human crumbling under a fire. Choice *A* is a simile and does not utilize alliteration or the use of consistent consonant sounds for effect. Choice *C* is a metaphor and does not utilize alliteration. Choice *D* describes neither alliteration nor personification.

39. B: The correct answer is an infectious disease. By reading context, all other options can be eliminated since the author restates zymosis as disease.

40. D: A *rookery* is a colony of breeding birds. Although *rookery* could mean Choice *A*, houses in a slum area, it does not make sense in this context. Choices *B* and *C* are both incorrect, as this is not a place for hunters to trade tools or for wardens to trade stories.

41. A: The topic of the passage is Caribbean island destinations. The *topic* of the passage can be described in a one- or two-word phrase. Remember, when paraphrasing a passage, it is important to include the topic. Paraphrasing is when one puts a passage into his or her own words.

42. C: Family or adult-only resorts and activities are supporting details in this passage. *Supporting details* are details that help readers better understand the main idea. They answer questions such as who, what, where, when, why, or how. In this question, cruises and local events are not discussed in the passage, whereas family and adult-only resorts and activities support the main idea.

43. D: Choice *D* correctly summarizes Frost's theme of life's journey and the choices one makes. While Choice *A* can be seen as an interpretation, it is a literal one and is incorrect. Literal is not symbolic. Choice *B* presents the idea of good and evil as a theme, and the poem does not specify this struggle for the traveler. Choice *C* is a similarly incorrect answer. Love is not the theme.

44. C: There are 20 lines in this poem. You can see the number of lines to the right of the poem (it goes to 20), or you can count the lines individually.

45. A: This poem is made up of one stanza. Lines in poems are the individual lines that break from one line to the next. Stanzas are groups of lines. If this poem had another stanza, we would see a space between a group of lines, almost like a paragraph. This poem has only one block of lines.

46. A: There is only one traveler in the poem. We see this in the line "And be one traveler, long I stood." This indicates that the speaker is alone and traveling without a partner.

47. B: The time of day in the poem is morning. The line we see this in says, "And both that morning equally lay." This question relies on how carefully the passage was read.

48. B: The traveler took the second road. We see the traveler unsure at first about whether to take the first or second road. After they choose the second road, they contemplate saving "the first for another day," but they never take the first road in the poem.

Vocabulary

1. C: The blood vessels that carry deoxygenated blood back to the heart are called *veins*. *Capillaries* are where arteries and veins meet to exchange oxygen and carbon dioxide at the tissue level. *Arteries* carry oxygenated blood away from the heart to the tissues of the body. *Ventricles* are a type of blood-pumping chamber in the heart, although there are ventricles in the brain as well that serve a different purpose.

2. D: The patient is displaying *displacement*, in which he is taking his negative feelings towards the doctor and expressing them towards the nurse aide, unfairly. *Reaction formation* is when the person feels negatively but reacts positively. *Intellectualization* is when a person focuses on minute details of the situation rather than coping with the negative emotions associated with it. *Undoing* is when the person has done something wrong and acts excessively in the opposite way to "redeem" themselves of their prior wrong-doing.

3. B: A *teacher* provides instruction and information to an individual or group of individuals. An *instructor* functions in the same capacity, that is, in the practice of teaching. A *pupil* is one being taught or instructed. A *survivor* is one who continues through an experience which may or may not refer to the experience of a pupil or student. A *dictator* is one who dictates or pronounces with authority but does not necessarily explain as a teacher or instructor would.

4. A: The chest pain as described in this patient's situation most likely is cardiac in origin, so the patient could be experiencing a *myocardial infarction*, or heart attack. Chest pain associated with *gastroesophageal reflux* is more often described as a burning sensation, without the other symptoms described. *Pneumonia* and *pleuritis* may both cause the patient to have a different type of chest pain, in which a sharp, stabbing sensation is felt upon breathing.

5. A: *Reconnaissance* is a noun that means preliminary research or surveying. It is also used in a military context where a *reconnaissance* is the surveying or observation to obtain information for strategic planning or to locate an enemy.

6. C: Something *ineffable* cannot be described with words. It often is used in connection to something so impressive, emotional, or great. The heartwarming feelings of a family reuniting after a parent has been deployable may be said to be *ineffable.*

7. C: Someone that is described as *gregarious* is social and talkative. *Meek* is more of an antonym because it means quiet and submissive.

8. A: *Caustic* is an adjective that is often used in the chemical context to describe a substance that is corrosive or able to burn tissues. In this way, it is typically an acidic and abrasive chemical. However, it can also be used to describe a person's demeanor, which is bitterly sarcastic or scathing.

9. C: This type of seizure with muscle rigidity, convulsions, and unconsciousness is called a *grand mal* seizure. A *myoclonic* seizure only involves one part of the body making jerking movements. An *absence* seizure involves a brief loss of consciousness where the patient may stare off into space. A *tonic* seizure is characterized by rigidity and stiffness of the muscles.

10. D: The patient is most likely experiencing a stroke, as evidenced by the difficulty with speech and facial drooping. *Meningitis* is an inflammation of the meninges and does not fit the description of symptoms here. A *migraine* is a severe headache that can sometimes mimic stroke symptoms but is less severe. A stroke should be suspected until it is proven otherwise in order to get the patient timely and effective treatment. A *seizure* is characterized by muscle rigidity, convulsions, and loss of consciousness.

11. A: This patient is at risk for *hypoglycemia*, or a blood sugar less than 60mg/dL due to the missed meals and perhaps missed regular insulin and anti-diabetic medication dosages. A disruption in a diabetic patient's schedule can lead to hypoglycemia and the nurse aide should be vigilant in monitoring the patient's intake. *Diabetic ketoacidosis* is a result of too much blood sugar, or hyperglycemia. A *diabetic coma* is possible in both the cases of hyper- and hypoglycemia, but the patient is still conscious, so that rules that option out. *Hyperglycemia* is a blood sugar greater than 200mg/dL and is not likely, since this patient has not had any oral intake.

12. A: Someone that is *obtuse* is unintelligent or slow-witted. They might be described as ignorant or dense. In geometry, it refers to an angle greater than 90 degrees and less than 180 degrees, but this is a different usage of the word.

13. C: A patient who is *somnolent* can be described as sleepy, only arousing to verbal stimuli but returning to sleep when the stimuli is stopped. *Delirium* is characterized by confusion and agitation and has to do with the patient's ability to pay attention. *Coma* is a state in which the patient cannot be aroused at all, either by verbal or painful stimuli. *Stupor* refers to someone who is sleeping that only arouses to painful stimuli.

14. B: The medical term for coughing up blood in the sputum is *hemoptysis*. *Hematopoiesis* is the process of creating new blood cells in the body. *Hematemesis* is when there is blood in the vomitus. *Hematochezia* refers to rectal bleeding.

15. C: *Sordid* means filthy, vile, or squalid. *Semantic* means referring to the meaning of words or language. *Surly* can mean either threatening in appearance or crabby (in terms of mood).

16. A: *Bereavement* may present as many different physical conditions and can be diagnosed by completing a thorough history. *Stroke* often presents as deficits on one side of the body. *Anorexia nervosa* presents with decreased appetite along with signs of malnutrition. *MI (myocardial infarction)* often presents with tingling or pain in the left arm or jaw and chest pressure or pain.

17. C: Alternative medications are often ordered in place of antispasmodics for treatment of urinary incontinence due to side effects of excessive thirst.

18. A: To *solicit* is to ask for something, often with the goal of obtaining something from someone else. *Solicitation* is the noun that is derived from the term; it refers to the act of asking for something. Sometimes, homes or businesses will post a notice that "no solicitation is allowed," meaning no one is to knock on the door trying to sell something, asking for signatures in support of a cause, etc.

19. C: *Venous* ulcers are commonly found between the knees and ankles. *Arterial* ulcers are located at the end of the toe on pressure points or in non-healing wounds. *Neuropathic* ulcers are found on the toes and sides of the feet. *Staging* applies to all types of ulcers and is dependent upon size, tunneling, and other factors.

20. A: *Isometric* exercises are done against resistance without moving a joint. *Isotonic* exercise moves the joint, *isokinetic* exercise uses a machine, and *plyometric* exercise uses a combination of stretching followed by contraction.

21. C: Tendons connect muscle to bone. Ligaments connect bone to bone. Both are made of dense, fibrous connective tissue (primary Type 1 collagen) to give strength. However, tendons are more organized, especially in the long axis direction like muscle fibers themselves, and they have more collagen. This arrangement makes more sense because muscles have specific orientations of their fibers, so they contract in somewhat predictable directions. Ligaments are less organized and more of a woven pattern because bone connections are not as organized as bundles or muscle fibers, so ligaments must have strength in multiple directions to protect against injury.

22. C: The axial skeleton includes the bones of the skull and face (so the mandible, or jaw bone is included), the ribs, the vertebral column (so the atlas, which is the name of the first cervical bone, is included), the sternum, and the hyoid. The bones of the shoulder girdle, clavicles, pelvis, and limbs are considered the bones the comprise the appendicular skeleton. Therefore, the illium, a bone of the pelvis, is not part of the axial skeleton.

23. A: The sternum is medial to the deltoid because it is much closer (typically right on) the midline of the body, while the deltoid is lateral at the shoulder cap. Superficial means that a structure is closer to the body surface and posterior means that it falls behind something else. For example, skin is superficial to bone and the kidneys are posterior to the rectus abdominus.

24. D: The outermost layer of the skin, the epidermis, consists of *epithelial* cells. This layer of skin is dead, as it has no blood vessels. *Osteoclasts* are cells that make up bones. Notice the prefix *Osteo-* which means bone. *Connective* tissue macrophage cells can be found in a variety of places, and *dendritic* cells are part of the lymphatic system.

25. A: The Haversian system in compact bone is composed of embedded blood vessels, lymph vessels, and nerve bundles that span the interior of the bone from one end to the other. Volkmann's canals extend from the central canal to the periosteum to deliver materials to peripheral osteocytes. Choice *C* is describing the lamellae, which are concentric circles that surround the central Haversian canal with gaps between them called lacunae where osteocytes are embedded.

26. C: *Cubital,* in terms of body regions, refers to the elbow. For example, the inner elbow area where blood draws are often collected is called the antecubital space. The shoulder region is referred to as the *acromial* area.

27. C: Eosinophils, like neutrophils, basophils, and mast cells, are a type of leukocyte in a class called granulocytes. They are found underneath mucous membranes in the body and they primarily secrete destructive enzymes and defend against multicellular parasites like worms. Choice *A* describes basophils and mast cells, and Choices *B* and *D* describe neutrophils. Unlike neutrophils, which are aggressive phagocytic cells, eosinophils have low phagocytic activity.

28. A: *Keratin* is a structural protein, and it is the primary constituent of things like hair and nails. Choice *B* is incorrect; *antigens* are immune proteins that help fight disease. Choice *C* is incorrect because *channel proteins* are transport proteins that help move molecules into and out of a cell. Lastly, Choice *D* is incorrect because *actin,* like myosin, is a motor protein because it is involved in the process of muscle contraction.

29. B: Deep. The dermis is the deeper layer of skin under the more superficial epidermis.

30. C: A professional who draws blood. An x-ray technician takes x-rays, a prosthetist makes artificial limbs, and a psychologist, social worker, or therapist counsels patients.

31. C: Regress. *Rescind* means to revoke or repeal. It often is used in relation to an agreement or law. *Digress* means to temporarily deviate from the main topic when speaking or writing (for example, telling a story that is just somewhat related to the main point). *Diverge* is to fork or separate from the main path or road.

32. C: The shoulder. The acromion process is a bony protrusion on the scapula that extends laterally toward the shoulder joint. The acromioclavicular ligament connects the acromion process with the clavicle.

33. B: Expressionless. Glassy eyes, like a doll's, are shiny and empty; they are expressionless. Someone with glassy eyes may have a fixed stare. Different conditions, such as severe dehydration and cholera, can cause glassy eyes.

34. A: Flush. Though *flush* has several definitions, in the context of the provided sentence, it means to align in a smooth, consistent way, forming an unbroken surface. It's important for braces, for example AFOs (ankle foot orthoses), to be flush with the skin. Otherwise, friction will occur between the skin and the brace where it contacts a prominence and cause blistering or skin breakdown.

35. C: To supply nerves to. For example, the radial nerve innervates the extensors in the upper arm, such as the triceps.

36. A: Amputation. Gangrene is localized dead or necrotic tissue, which can be caused by insufficient blood flow. For example, a toe may be affected by gangrene in someone with poorly controlled, advanced diabetes.

37. C: Exigent. *Lenient* means permissive and easy-going, to *extoll* is to praise, and *lackadaisical* means apathetic or lazy.

38. D: Language impairment. *Aphasia* is a loss in the ability to express or understand speech, so it is language impairment. It is often caused by brain damage, whether due to a stroke, TBI, or other cause. An inability to recognize things is *agnosia*.

39. C: Nothing by mouth. NPO comes from the Latin *nil per os,* which means nothing by mouth. Do not resuscitate is abbreviated DNR.

40. A: Dull. Something that is *jejune* is simplistic, naïve, or unoriginal.

41. A: Deficit. *Diffident* means shy or lacking in confidence. *Dearth* means scarcity, so it might be an attractive choice, but *deficit* is a better word in the context of the sentence. *Diffident* means obstinate or uncooperative.

42. D: Contradiction. A paradox often seems self-contradictory; something that is true yet doesn't follow what's expected or logical.

43. A: Lithe. While Choice *B, ballerina,* may be described as agile and graceful, the correct choice is the adjective that describes the movement, *lithe.*

44. B: Cyanosis. Cyanosis often results from an occlusion or circulation impairment, which causes an insufficient amount of oxygen to perfuse the tissues.

45. A: Respect. Someone who is venerated is respected and revered.

46. B: Mycosis. The prefix *myco-* means something related to fungus.

47. C: Uremia. *Anuria* is no urine production, *nocturia* is nighttime urination, and *polyrurea* refers to abnormally large volumes of urine.

48. B: A sustained muscle contraction. A single nerve impulse initiates a muscle twitch, whereas when many impulses sum together, the muscle contraction is sustained in what is called tetanus. Tetanus occurs with repeated stimulation without a break for the muscle to relax.

49. A: Spatial awareness of the body. The body has sensory receptors, called proprioceptors, which help the body sense and respond to position and movement.

50. C: To refrain from something. For example, someone who chooses to *abstain* from alcohol does not drink alcohol.

Grammar

1. C: The clause *that there is an afterlife* is the noun telling us *what belief.* Choice *A* is incorrect because *the belief that* is not a clause; it has no verb. Choice *B* is incorrect because *is a personal choice* is not a clause because it has no subject. Choice *D* is incorrect because *is an afterlife* is not a clause because it has no subject.

2. B: The clause *who loves to ride bikes* is a restrictive adjective clause modifying the noun *boy.* Choice *A* is incorrect because *a boy who loves* is a phrase not a clause. Choice *C* is incorrect because *to ride bikes* is an infinitive phrase and does not have a subject. Choice *D* is incorrect because *gets plenty of exercise* is not a clause; it has no subject.

3. D: The adverbial clause *unless you are too tired* modifies the verb *want*. Choice *A* is incorrect because *I want to work in the garden* is an independent clause. Choice *B* is incorrect because *in the garden* has no subject and is a prepositional phrase. Choice *C* is incorrect because *are too tired* is not a clause because it has no subject.

4. C: A noun phrase is a noun and all of its modifiers; in this case, *long* and *black* are adjectives modifying the noun *limousine* and *the* is an article modifying *limousine*. Choice *A* is incorrect because it identifies the compound subject of the sentence. Choice *B* is incorrect because it includes the verb *rode*. Choice *D* is incorrect because it includes a subject and a verb, and phrases do not have both.

5. B: Choice *B* is correct because the idea of the original sentences is Armani getting lost while walking through Paris. Choice *A* is incorrect because it replaces third person with second person. Choice *C* is incorrect because the word *should* indicates an obligation to get lost. Choice *D* is incorrect because it is not specific to the original sentence but instead makes a generalization about getting lost.

6. C: There is no gerund phrase in the sentence. Choice *A* is incorrect because *swimming several laps* is a gerund phrase serving as the noun subject of the sentence. Choice *B* is incorrect because *using the flippers* is a gerund phrase serving as the noun object of the sentence. Choice *D* is incorrect because *learning to swim* is a gerund phrase serving as the noun subject of the sentence.

7. A: *My second cousin* is a nonessential appositive phrase renaming *Carrie Fisher*. Because it is nonessential, it is set off by commas in the sentence. Choice *B* is incorrect because *Harrison Ford* is an essential appositive explaining which actor is being discussed. Choice *C* is incorrect because there is no appositive phrase in the sentence. Choice *D* is incorrect because *Star Wars* is an essential appositive explaining which movie is being discussed.

8. B: *The fire crackling* is an absolute phrase that includes a participle following a noun and has nothing to do with the rest of the sentence but cannot stand alone as its own sentence. Choice *A* is incorrect because *going camping in the forest* is a gerund phrase serving as the noun object of the sentence. Choice *C* is incorrect because *hot cocoa and coffee* is a nonessential appositive phrase renaming *the best drinks*. Choice *D* is incorrect because *for school-age children* is a prepositional phrase.

9. C: Choice *C* is correct because it shows that Phoenix buried his cat with her favorite toys after she died, which is true of the original statement. Although Choices *A*, *B*, and *D* mention a backyard, the meanings of these choices are skewed. Choice *A* says that Phoenix buried his cat alive, which is incorrect. Choice *B* says his cat died in the backyard, which we do not know to be true. Choice *D* says Phoenix buried his cat after he buried her toys, which is also incorrect.

10. D: Choice *D* is correct because it expresses the sentiment of a moment of joy bringing tears to one's eyes as one sees a sunset while in a helicopter. Choice *A* is incorrect because it implies that the person was outside of the helicopter watching it from afar. Choice *B* is incorrect because the original sentence does not portray the sunset *flying up* into the sky. Choice *C* is incorrect because, while the helicopter may have been facing the sunset, this is not the reason that tears were in the speaker's eyes.

11. A: Answer Choice *A* uses the best, most concise word choice. Choice *B* uses the pronoun *that* to refer to people instead of *who*. *Choice C* incorrectly uses the preposition *with*. Choice *D* uses the preposition *for* and the additional word *any*, making the sentence wordy and less clear.

12. B: Choice *B* uses the best choice of words to create a subordinate and independent clause. In Choice *A*, *because* makes it seem like this is the reason I enjoy working from home, which is incorrect. In Choice

C, the word *maybe* creates two independent clauses, which are not joined properly with a comma. Choice *D* uses *with*, which does not make grammatical sense.

13. B: The original sentence focuses on how politicians are using the student debt issue to their advantage, so Choice *B* is the best answer choice. Choice *A* says politicians want students' votes but suggests that it is the reason for student loan debt, which is incorrect. Choice *C* shifts the focus to voters, when the sentence is really about politicians. Choice *D* is vague and doesn't best restate the original meaning of the sentence.

14. A: This answer best matches the meaning of the original sentence, which states that seasoned runners offer advice to new runners because they have complaints of injuries. Choice *B* may be true, but it doesn't mention the complaints of injuries by new runners. Choice *C* may also be true, but it does not match the original meaning of the sentence. Choice *D* does not make sense in the context of the sentence.

15. D: To create parallelism, make both verbal gerunds. Choice *A* is incorrect. *Chewing* is a gerund and *to play* is an infinitive. Choice *B* is incorrect. *To chew* is an infinitive and *playing* is a gerund. Choice *C* is incorrect. *To chew* and *to play* are both infinitives, but they do not match with the verb *enjoy*.

16. B: Both verb phrases are introduced with the word *who*, creating parallelism. Choice *A* is incorrect. The introductory words for the verb phrases do not match. Choice *C* is incorrect. The introductory words for the verb phrases do not match and the word *that* would modify an object, not a person. Use *who* for a person. Choice *D* is incorrect. The word *that* in the sentence should be used to modify an object not a person, and the clown is a person.

17. A: The linking verbs *have been* are the same in both verb phrases, creating parallelism. Choice *B* is incorrect. *Have been traveling* does not match with *were sightseeing*. Choice *C* is incorrect. Again, *were traveling* does not match with *have been sightseeing*. Choice *D* is incorrect. The tenses of the verbs do not match. *Have been traveling* does not match with *they are sightseeing*.

18. D: To make *the building was sturdy and solid* subordinate to *the building crumbled in the earthquake,* create a dependent clause with the less important piece of information. Choice *A* is incorrect. It is two independent clauses joined with a semicolon and neither piece of information is subordinate to the other. Choice *B* is incorrect. This sentence implies that the building was still sturdy and solid after crumbling in the earthquake because the word *although* is misplaced. Choice *C* is incorrect because, even though it is a grammatically correct sentence, neither piece of information is subordinate to the other.

19. A: In this example, a colon is correctly used to introduce a series of items. Choice *B* places an unnecessary comma before the word *because*. A comma is not needed before the word *because* when it introduces a dependent clause at the end of a sentence and provides necessary information to understand the sentence. Choice *C* is incorrect because it uses a semi-colon instead of a comma to join a dependent clause and an independent clause. Choice *D* is incorrect because it uses a colon in place of a comma and coordinating conjunction to join two independent clauses.

20. B: Choice *B* correctly uses the contraction for *you are* as the subject of the sentence, and it correctly uses the possessive pronoun *your* to indicate ownership of the jacket. It also correctly uses the adverb *there*, indicating place. Choice *A* is incorrect because it reverses the possessive pronoun *your* and the contraction for *you are*. It also uses the possessive pronoun *their* instead of the adverb *there*. Choice *C* is incorrect because it reverses *your* and *you're* and uses the contraction for *they are* in place of the adverb *there*. Choice *D* incorrectly uses the possessive pronoun *their* instead of the adverb *there*.

21. A: Only two of these suffixes, *–ize* and *–en*, can be used to form verbs, so *B* and *D* are incorrect. Those choices create adjectives. The suffix *–ize* means "to convert or turn into." The suffix *–en* means "to become." Because this sentence is about converting ideas into money, money + *–ize* or *monetize* is the most appropriate word to complete the sentence, so *C* is incorrect.

22. B: In Choice *B,* the word *Uncle* should not be capitalized, because it is not functioning as a proper noun. If the word named a specific uncle, such as *Uncle Jerry*, then it would be considered a proper noun and should be capitalized. Choice *A* correctly capitalizes the proper noun *East Coast*, and does not capitalize *winter*, which functions as a common noun in the sentence. Choice *C* correctly capitalizes the name of a specific college course, which is considered a proper noun. Choice *D* correctly capitalizes the proper noun *Jersey Shore*.

23. C: In Choice *C, avid* is functioning as an adjective that modifies the word photographer. *Avid* describes the photographer Julia Robinson's style. The words *time* and *photographer* are functioning as nouns, and the word *capture* is functioning as a verb in the sentence. Other words functioning as adjectives in the sentence include, *local, business*, and *spare*, as they all describe the nouns they precede.

24. A: Choice *A* is correctly punctuated because it uses a semicolon to join two independent clauses that are related in meaning. Each of these clauses could function as an independent sentence. Choice *B* is incorrect because the conjunction is not preceded by a comma. A comma and conjunction should be used together to join independent clauses. Choice *C* is incorrect because a comma should only be used to join independent sentences when it also includes a coordinating conjunction such as *and* or *so*. Choice *D* does not use punctuation to join the independent clauses, so it is considered a fused (same as a run-on) sentence.

25. C: Choice *C* is a compound sentence because it joins two independent clauses with a comma and the coordinating conjunction *and*. The sentences in Choices B and D include one independent clause and one dependent clause, so they are complex sentences, not compound sentences. The sentence in Choice *A* has both a compound subject, *Alex and Shane*, and a compound verb, *spent and took*, but the entire sentence itself is one independent clause.

26. C: The suffix *-fy* means to make, cause, or cause to have. Choices A, B, and D are incorrect because they show meanings of other suffixes. Choice *A* shows the meaning of the suffix *-ous*. Choice *B* shows the meaning of the suffix *–ist*, and choice D shows the meaning of the suffix *-age*.

27. A: *After* and *then* are transitional words that indicate time or position. Choice *B* is incorrect because the words *at, with,* and *to* are used as prepositions in this sentence, not transitions. Choice *C* is incorrect because the words *had* and *took* are used as verbs in this sentence. In Choice *D, a* and *the* are used as articles in the sentence.

28. C: Choice *C* is a compound sentence because it joins two independent clauses—*The baby was sick* and *I decided to stay home from work*—with a comma and the coordinating conjunction *so*. Choices A, B, and D, are all simple sentences, each containing one independent clause with a complete subject and predicate. Choices A and D each contain a compound subject, or more than one subject, but they are still simple sentences that only contain one independent clause. Choice *B* contains a compound verb (more than one verb), but it's still a simple sentence.

29. A: Choice *A* includes all of the words functioning as nouns in the sentence. Choice *B* is incorrect because it includes the words *final* and *academic,* which are functioning as adjectives in this sentence. The word *he* makes Choice *C* incorrect because it is a pronoun. This example also includes the word *library*, which can function as a noun, but is functioning as an adjective modifying the word *databases* in this sentence. Choice *D* is incorrect because it leaves out the proper noun *Robert*.

30. C: The simple subject of this sentence, the word *lots*, is plural. It agrees with the plural verb form *were*. Choice *A* is incorrect, because the simple subject *there*, referring to the two constellations, is considered plural. It does not agree with the singular verb form *is*. In Choice *B*, the singular subject *four*, does not agree with the plural verb form *needs*. In Choice *D* the plural subject *everyone* does not agree with the singular verb form *have*.

31. B: *Excellent* and *walking* are adjectives modifying the noun *tours*. *Rich* is an adjective modifying the noun *history*, and *brotherly* is an adjective modifying the noun *love*. Choice *A* is incorrect because all of these words are functioning as nouns in the sentence. Choice *C* is incorrect because all of these words are functioning as verbs in the sentence. Choice *D* is incorrect because all of these words are considered prepositions, not adjectives.

32. C: The dependent adjective clause *cute and cuddly* does not modify *the children*, it modifies *teddy bears*. The modifier is misplaced. Choice *A* does not contain a misplaced modifier. It is a grammatically correct independent clause. Choice *B* does not have a misplaced modifier. It is a grammatically correct compound sentence with two independent clauses joined with a semicolon. Choice *D* does not have a misplaced modifier. The modifier *cute and cuddly* correctly modifies *teddy bears*. The sentence is grammatically correct.

33. B: *Dissatisfied* and *accommodations* are both spelled correctly in Choice *B*. These are both considered commonly misspelled words. One or both words are spelled incorrectly in choices A, C, and D.

34. B: Choice *B* is an imperative sentence because it issues a command. In addition, it ends with a period, and an imperative sentence must end in a period or exclamation mark. Choice *A* is a declarative sentence that states a fact and ends with a period. Choice *C* is an exclamatory sentence that shows strong emotion and ends with an exclamation point. Choice *D* is an interrogative sentence that asks a question and ends with a question mark.

35. A: It is necessary to put a comma between the date and the year. It is also required to put a comma between the day of the week and the month. Choice *B* is incorrect because it is missing the comma between the day and year. Choice *C* is incorrect because it adds an unnecessary comma between the month and date. Choice *D* is missing the necessary comma between day of the week and the month.

36. D: To create parallelism, make both verbal gerunds. Choice *A* is incorrect. *Chewing* is a gerund and *to play* is an infinitive. Choice *B* is incorrect. *To chew* is an infinitive and *playing* is a gerund. Choice *C* is incorrect. *To chew* and *to play* are both infinitives, but they do not match with the verb *enjoy*.

37. D: In Choice *D*, the word function is a noun. While the word *function* can also act as a verb, in this particular sentence it is acting as a noun as the object of the preposition *at*. Choices A and B are incorrect because the word *function* cannot be used as an adjective or adverb.

38. C: Cacti is the correct plural form of the word *cactus*. Choice A (*tomatos*) includes an incorrect spelling of the plural of *tomato*. Both choice B (*analysis*) and choice D (*criterion*) are incorrect because they are in singular form. The correct plural form for these choices would be *criteria* and analyses.

39. B: Quotation marks are used to indicate something someone said. The example sentences feature a direct quotation that requires the use of double quotation marks. Also, the end punctuation, in this case a question mark, should always be contained within the quotation marks. Choice A is incorrect because there is an unnecessary period after the quotation mark. Choice C is incorrect because it uses single quotation marks, which are used for a quote within a quote. Choice D is incorrect because it places the punctuation outside of the quotation marks.

40. D: The prefix *trans* means across, beyond, over. Choices A, B, and C are incorrect because they are the meanings of other prefixes. Choice A is a meaning of the prefix *de*. Choice B is the meaning of the prefix *omni*. Choice C is one of the meanings of the prefix *pro*. The example words are helpful in determining the meaning of *trans*. All of the example words—*transfer, transact, translation, transport*—indicate something being *across, beyond,* or *over* something else. For example, *translation* refers to text going across languages. If no example words were given, you could think of words starting with *trans* and then compare their meanings to try to determine a common definition.

41. D: In choice D, the word *part* functions as an adjective that modifies the word *Irish*. Choices A and C are incorrect because the word *part* functions as a noun in these sentences. Choice B is incorrect because the word *part* functions as a verb.

42. C: *All of Shannon's family and friends* is the complete subject because it includes who or what is doing the action in the sentence as well as the modifiers that go with it. Choice A is incorrect because it only includes the simple subject of the sentence. Choices B and D are incorrect because they only include part of the complete subject.

43. D: Choice D directly addresses the reader, so it is in second person point of view. This is an imperative sentence since it issues a command; imperative sentences have an *understood you* as the subject. Choice A uses first person pronouns *I* and *my*. Choices B and C are incorrect because they use third person point of view.

44. A: The word *prodigious* is defined as very impressive, amazing, or large. In this sentence, the meaning can be drawn from the words *they became nervous about climbing its distant peak*, as this would be an appropriate reaction upon seeing a very large peak that's far in the distance. Choices B, C, and D do not accurately define the word *prodigious*, so they are incorrect.

45. D: Choice D correctly places a hyphen after the prefix *ex* to join it to the word *husband.* Words that begin with the prefixes *great, trans, ex, all,* and *self,* require a hyphen. Choices A and C place hyphens in words where they are not needed. *Beagle mix* would only require a hyphen if coming before the word *Henry*, since it would be serving as a compound adjective in that instance. Choice B contains hyphens that are in the correct place but are formatted incorrectly since they include spaces between the hyphens and the surrounding words.

46. C: Choice C is correct because quotation marks should be used for the title of a short work such as a poem. Choices A, B, and D are incorrect because the titles of novels, films, and newspapers should be placed in italics, not quotation marks.

47. A: This question focuses on the correct usage of the commonly confused word pairs of *it's/its* and *then/than*. *It's* is a contraction for *it is* or *it has*. *Its* is a possessive pronoun. The word *than* shows comparison between two things. *Then* is an adverb that conveys time. Choice *C* correctly uses *it's* and *than*. *It's* is a contraction for *it has* in this sentence, and *than* shows comparison between *work* and *rest*. None of the other answers choices use both of the correct words.

48. C: The original sentence states that firefighting is dangerous, making it necessary for firefighters to wear protective gear. The portion of the sentence that needs to be rewritten focuses on the gear, not the dangers, of firefighting. Choices *A*, *B*, and *D* all discuss the danger, not the gear, so *C* is the correct answer.

49. D: The original sentence states that though the sites are popular, they can be dangerous for teens, so *D* is the best choice. Choice *A* does state that there is danger, but it doesn't identify teens and limits it to just one site. Choice *B* repeats the statement from the beginning of the sentence, and Choice *C* says the sites are used too much, which is not the point made in the original sentence.

50. A: The affix *circum–* originates from Latin and means *around or surrounding*. It is also related to other round words, such as circle and circus. The rest of the choices do not relate to the affix *circum–* and are therefore incorrect.

Biology

1. B: The structure exclusively found in eukaryotic cells is the nucleus. Animal, plant, fungi, and protist cells are all eukaryotic. DNA is contained within the nucleus of eukaryotic cells, and they also have membrane-bound organelles that perform complex intracellular metabolic activities. Prokaryotic cells (archae and bacteria) do not have a nucleus or other membrane-bound organelles and are less complex than eukaryotic cells.

2. A: The Golgi apparatus is designed to tag, package, and ship out proteins destined for other cells or locations. The centrioles typically play a large role only in cell division when they ratchet the chromosomes from the mitotic plate to the poles of the cell. The mitochondria are involved in energy production and are the powerhouses of the cell. The cell structure responsible for cellular storage, digestion and waste removal is the lysosome. Lysosomes are like recycle bins. They are filled with digestive enzymes that facilitate catabolic reactions to regenerate monomers.

3. C: A male moose with horns that enable him to reduce competition for mating. Choices *A* and *D* (elephant and monkey) are not caused by genes. These are learned behaviors from other animals. Choice *B* (smelly dog) is actually a detriment because the dog will be less likely to mate, so she will not pass on her smelly genes.

4. D: All of the above. Let's label *R* as the right-handed allele and *r* as the left-handed allele. Esther has to have the combination rr since she's left-handed. She had to get at least one recessive allele from each parent. So, mom could either be Rr or rr (right-handed or left-handed), and dad can also be Rr or rr. As long as each parent carries one recessive allele, it is possible that Esther is left-handed. Therefore, all answer choices are possible.

5. A: Organ: Heart. Blank #1 is tissue and blank #2 is organ, so Choices *C* and *D* are automatically incorrect. Blood vessels (*B*) are a type of smooth muscle tissue. The heart is an organ.

The following image is for question 10.

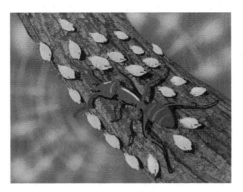

6. C: Mutualism. In the ant-aphid case, both organisms benefit, as the ants are getting food and the aphids are getting protection. Competition (*A*) is when organisms want the same thing (food, water, shelter, space), which is clearly not the case here. Parasitism (*B*) involves one organism getting hurt in the relationship at the expense of the other, while commensalism (*D*) involves an organism that is benefited connected to an indifferent party.

7. D: All living and nonliving things in an area. Choice *C* (all the organisms in a food web) describes feeding relationships and not symbiosis. Choice *B* (rocks, soil, and atmosphere in an area) includes nonliving factors in an ecosystem. Choice *A*, one organism, is too small to be considered an ecosystem.

8. C: Oxygen. Water (*A*) is a reactant that gets sucked up by the roots. Carbon dioxide (*D*) is a reactant that goes into the stomata, and sunlight (*B*) inputs energy into the reaction in order to create the high-energy sugar.

9. C: Breaking down food to release energy. Breathing (*B*) is not cellular respiration; breathing is an action that takes place at the organism level with the respiratory system. Making high-energy sugars (*A*) is photosynthesis, not cellular respiration. Perspiration (*D*) is sweating, and has nothing to do with cellular respiration.

10. D: Algae can perform photosynthesis. One indicator that a plant is able to perform photosynthesis is the color green. Plants with the pigment chlorophyll are able to absorb the warmer colors of the light spectrum, but are unable to absorb green. That's why they appear green. Choices *A* and *C* are types of fungi, and are therefore not able to perform photosynthesis. Fungi obtain energy from food in their environment. Choice *B*, ant, is also unable to perform photosynthesis, since it is an animal.

11. D: The solar waves from the sun warm the earth. Many of the waves are meant to reflect back off of the atmosphere to keep the earth warm, and the rest of the waves are meant to reflect back out into space through the atmosphere. This is known as the greenhouse effect. However, when the atmosphere has become too dense (polluted by gases), the waves meant to escape are trapped and re-radiate in the earth's atmosphere, causing an overall warming of the climate, known as global warming.

12. D: Fungi. Choice *A* (the sun) is not even a living thing. Grass (*B*) is a producer, and the frog (*C*) is a consumer. The fungi break down dead organisms and are the only decomposer shown.

13. B: Grasshopper. An herbivore is an organism that eats only plants, and that's the grasshopper's niche in this particular food chain. Grass (*A*) is a producer, the frog (*C*) is a consumer, and the fungi (*D*) is a decomposer.

14. D: Human gametes each contain 23 chromosomes. This is referred to as haploid—half the number of the original germ cell (46). Germ cells are diploid precursors of the haploid egg and sperm. Meiosis has two major phases, each of which is characterized by sub-phases similar to mitosis. In Meiosis I, the DNA of the parent cell is duplicated in interphase, just like in mitosis. Starting with prophase I, things become a little different. Two homologous chromosomes form a tetrad, cross over, and exchange genetic content. Each shuffled chromosome of the tetrad migrates to the cell's poles, and two haploid daughter cells are formed. In Meiosis II, each daughter undergoes another division more similar to mitosis (with the exception of the fact that there is no interphase), resulting in four genetically-different cells, each with only ½ of the chromosomal material of the original germ cell.

15. A: The crossing over, or rearrangement of chromosomal sections in tetrads during meiosis, results in each gamete having a different combination of alleles than other gametes. *B* is incorrect because the presence of a Y chromosome determines gender. *C* is incorrect because it is improper separation in anaphase, not recombination, that causes non-disjunction. *D* is incorrect because transcription is an entirely different process involved in protein expression.

16. D: Both steps of photosynthesis usually occur during daylight because even though the Calvin cycle is not dependent on light energy, it *is* dependent upon the ATP and NADPH produced by the light reactions. This is because that energy can be invested into bonds to create high-energy sugars. For each G3P molecule produced, the Calvin cycle requires the investment of nine ATP molecules and six NADPH molecules.

17. A: The net products of anaerobic glycolysis from one six-carbon glucose molecule are 2 three-carbon pyruvate molecules; 2 reduced nicotinamide adenine dinucleotide (NADH) molecules, which are created when the electron carrier oxidized nicotinamide adenine dinucleotide (NAD+) peels off two electrons and a hydrogen atom; and 2 ATP molecules. Glycolysis requires two ATP molecules to drive the process forward, and since the gross end product is four ATP molecules, the net is 2 ATP molecules.

18. C: Glycolysis produces two pyruvate molecules per glucose molecule that gets broke down because glucose is a six-carbon sugar and pyruvate is a three-carbon sugar. Each pyruvate molecule oxidizes into a single acetyl-CoA molecule, which then enters the citric acid cycle. Therefore, two citric acid cycles can be completed per glucose molecule that initially entered glycolysis.

19. D: Oxidative phosphorylation includes two steps: the electron transport chain and chemiosmosis. These two processes help generate ATP molecules by transferring two electrons and a proton (H⁺) from each NADH and FADH₂ to channel proteins, pumping the hydrogen ions to the inner-membrane space using energy from the high-energy electrons to create a concentration gradient. In chemiosmosis, ATP synthase uses facilitated diffusion to deliver protons across the concentration gradient from the inner mitochondrial membrane to the matrix.

20. D: This question is looking for an analogous function animal cell structure to the plant cell structures of a plasmodesmata. Cell walls are only present in plant cells. The cell wall is made up of strong fibrous substances including cellulose and other polysaccharides, and protein. It is a layer outside of the plasma membrane, which protects the cell from mechanical damage and helps maintain the cell's shape. The plasmodesmata are found only in plant cells. They are cytoplasmic channels, or tunnels, that go through the cell wall and connect the cytoplasm of adjacent cells. The cell membrane is the animal cell analog to the plant cell wall. Like plasmodesmata, gap junctions in animal cells connect neighboring cells. They permit the transport of nutrients, ions, and other materials.

21. C: The mitochondrion is often called the powerhouse of the cell and is one of the most important structures for maintaining regular cell function. It is where aerobic cellular respiration occurs and where most of the cell's ATP is generated. The number of mitochondria in a cell varies greatly from organism to organism and from cell to cell. Cells that require more energy, like muscle cells, have more mitochondria.

22. A: Photosynthesis is the process of converting light energy into chemical energy, which is then stored in sugar and other organic molecules. The photosynthetic process takes place in the thylakoids inside chloroplast in plants. Chlorophyll is a green pigment that lives in the thylakoid membranes and absorbs photons from light.

23. B: Carbohydrates consist of sugars. The simplest sugar molecule is called a monosaccharide and has the molecular formula of CH_2O, or a multiple of that formula. Monosaccharides are important molecules for cellular respiration. Their carbon skeleton can also be used to rebuild new small molecules. Lipids are fats, proteins are formed via amino acids, and nucleic acid is found in DNA and RNA.

24. B: The secondary structure of a protein refers to the folds and coils that are formed by hydrogen bonding between the slightly charged atoms of the polypeptide backbone. The primary structure is the sequence of amino acids, similar to the letters in a long word. The tertiary structure is the overall shape of the molecule that results from the interactions between the side chains that are linked to the polypeptide backbone. The quaternary structure is the complete protein structure that occurs when a protein is made up of two or more polypeptide chains.

25. B: Models are representations of concepts that are impossible to experience directly, such as the 3D representation of DNA, so Choice *B* is correct. Choice *A* is incorrect because theories simply explain why things happen. Choice *C* is incorrect because laws describe how things happen. Choice *D* is false because an observation analyzes situations using human senses.

Chemistry

1. C: Conversion within the metric system is as simple as the movement of decimal points. The prefix *kilo-* means "one thousand," or three zeros, so the procedure to convert kilometers to the primary unit (meters) is to move the decimal point three units to the right. To get to centimeters, the decimal point must be moved an additional two places to the right: 0.78 → 78,000. Choice *A* is false because the decimal point has only been moved one place to right. Choice *B* is incorrect because the decimal point is moved two units in the wrong direction. Choice *D* is false because the decimal has only been moved three units to the right. The problem can also be solved by using the following conversion equation:

$$0.78 \text{km} \times \frac{1,000 \text{m}}{1 \text{km}} \times \frac{100 cm}{1 \text{m}} = 78,000 cm$$

2. B: The answer choices for this question are tricky. Converting to kilometers from miles will yield the choice 7.514 when using the conversion 1 mile = 1.609 km. However, because the value in miles is written to three significant figures, the answer choice should also yield a value in three significant figures, making 7.51 km the correct answer. Choices *C* and *D* could seem correct if someone flipped the conversion upside-down—that is, if they divided by 1.609 instead of multiplied by it.

$$4.67mi \times \frac{1.609km}{1mi} = 7.514 \ or \ 7.51$$

3. D: Isotones are atoms of different elements that have the same number of neutrons. Isotones will have different mass numbers, as will isotopes, which are atoms of the same element that have a different number of neutrons. Isobars are atoms that have the same number of nucleons (protons and neutrons), and therefore, they must have the same mass number.

4. D: Leading zeros (those present after a decimal) are never significant, while all non-zero digits are significant. Therefore, in the value 0.00067, the only significant figures are 6 and 7, so this value has only two significant figures, making Choice *D* correct. Choices *A*, *B*, and *C* assume that all or some of the zeros are significant, so these options are incorrect.

5. B: The set of results is close to the actual value of the acceleration due to gravity, making the results accurate. However, there is a different value recorded every time, so the results aren't precise, which makes Choice *B* the correct answer.

6. A: To find the mean, the sum of the values can be calculated and then divided by the number of values. To report the result to the appropriate number of significant figures, the number of significant figures in which the values were given must be identified. In this case, every value is given at two significant figures. When the values are added and divided by four, they yield a value of 6.425. However, because the values are given in two significant figures, then the answer is 6.4. Choices *B*, *C*, and *D* give an incorrect number of significant figures.

$$\frac{3.2 + 7.5 + 9.6 + 5.4}{4} = 6.4$$

7. D: Preparing a solution from a stock is simply a process of dilution by adding water to a certain amount of the stock. The amount of stock to use can be calculated using a formula and algebra:

$$V_S = \frac{M_D V_D}{M_S}$$

$$M_D = 1.5$$

$$V_D = 250ml$$

$$M_S = 12.0M$$

$$V_S = \frac{(1.5M)(250ml)}{12.0M} = 31.3ml$$

Because the given values are written to three significant figures, the answer should also be written in three significant figures, making Choice *D* the correct answer. The other answer choices are either incorrect values or reported to an incorrect number of significant figures.

8. B: When a solution is on the verge of—or in the process of—crystallization, it is called a *supersaturated* solution. This can also occur in a solution that seems stable, but if it is disturbed, the change can begin the crystallization process. To display the relationship between the mass of a solute that a solvent holds and a given temperature, a *solubility curve* is used. If a reading is on the solubility curve, the solvent is *saturated*; it is full and cannot hold more solute. If a reading is above the curve, the solvent is *supersaturated* and unstable from holding more solute than it should. If a reading is below the curve, the solvent is *unsaturated* and could hold more solute. Choices *A, C,* and *D* are all stable, whereas Choice *B* is unstable.

9. D: Electrons orbit the nucleus of the atom in atomic shells or orbitals. The first atomic shell, closest to the nucleus, can accommodate two electrons. The second atomic shell can hold a maximum of eight electrons, and the third atomic shell can also house a maximum of eight electrons. The tendency to want to fill the outer orbital completely (called the valence shell), or get rid of a sole electron in the valence shell, influences the degree to which an atom will readily form chemical bonds.

10 A: The metallic substance in an ionic bond often has low ionization energy. Coupled with the fact that the nonmetal has a high electron affinity, the metallic substance readily transfers an electron to the nonmetal. Choice *B* is incorrect because it is the nonmetallic substance, not the metallic one, that has a high electron affinity. Choice *C* is incorrect because ionic bonds are very strong. As such, ionic compounds have high melting and boiling points and are brittle and crystalline. Lastly, Choice *D* is incorrect because the reactions that forms ionic bonds are exothermic.

11. B: Electronegativity, or the measure of an atom's tendency to attract a bonding pair of electrons, doesn't quite follow the general trend in the Periodic table, so the order should be memorized. Although it generally increases diagonal from the lower left corner to the upper right corner, some of the common elements do not fall along this diagonal. The most electronegative element is fluorine. The following order of decreasing electronegativity should be helpful: F > O > Cl > N > Br > I > S > C > H > metals.

12. B: Unlike in ionic bonds where electrons are transferred between the bonding atoms, covalent bonds are formed when two atoms share electrons. The atoms in covalent compounds are bonded together because of the balance of attraction and repulsion between their protons and electrons. Two atoms can be joined by single, double, or triple covalent bonds. As the number of electrons that are shared increases, the length of the bond decreases because the atoms are held together more closely.

13. C: A solution is the term for a homogeneous mixture. A solution contains a solute (particle) dissolved in solvent (water). Solutions have the smallest solutes of the mixtures, dissolving very easily, and the solute is spread out evenly, or homogeneous. A colloid has medium-sized particles that are somewhat evenly spread out, but their major difference from solutions is that they have the Tyndall effect. Because their particles are larger, they will reflect light that will appear as a beam (Tyndall). The sun's rays are an example of Tyndall; the light is reflecting off of the large gas particles in the atmosphere. A suspension has very large particles that actually settle, creating a heterogeneous mixture.

14. B: Metallic compounds can conduct electricity by creating a current, which is formed by passing energy through the freely moving electrons. The electrons are shared by many metal cations are more fluid than those in ionic structures. They float around the bonded metals and form a sea of electrons. Lewis structures are not usually depicted for metallic structures because of this free-roaming ability of the electrons.

15. C: The qualitative definition of a gas or element's ionization energy is the amount of energy needed to remove a valence electron, or the one most loosely bound, from that substance and form a cation. Choice *A,* refers to atomic radius, Choice *B* refers to electronegativity, and Choice *D* refers to electron affinity. All four of these properties follow trends on the Periodic table.

16. C: Recall that the rate of a reaction is the measure of the change in concentration of the reactants or products over a certain period of time. When the reactants are in the gaseous state, increases in pressure increase the frequency of collisions between molecules because the compressed; therefore, the reaction rate increases because of these increased interactions and collisions. The reverse is true when pressure decreases; thus, the reaction rate decreases because there are fewer collisions between the gas molecules.

17. C: Equilibrium occurs when the rate of reactants forming products is equal to the rate of the products reverting back to the reactants. In equilibrium conditions, the concentration of reactants and products in the system doesn't change. The reaction shown is an example of heterogenous equilibrium because the substances are in different phases when equilibrium is reached. If, for example, the reactants and products were all gases, as in the conversion of sulphur dioxide to sulphur trioxide, and equilibrium is reached, it is considered homogenous equilibrium. There is not enough information provided in the equation to decide whether the system is in static or dynamic equilibrium because there is no indication about the whether the forward and reverse reactions are still occurring (dynamic equilibrium), or if all reactions have ceased (static equilibrium). Therefore, Choices A and B are incorrect.

18. C: Increasing temperature increases the rate of reactions due to increases in the kinetic energy of atoms and molecules. This increased movement results in increased collisions between reactants (with each other as well as with enzymes), which is the cause of the rate increase.

19. A: A chemical change alters the chemical makeup of the original object. When a piece of paper burns it cannot be returned to its original chemical makeup because it has formed new materials. Physical change refers to changing a substance's form, but not the composition of that substance. In physical science, "sedimentary change" and "potential change" are not terms used to describe any particular process.

20. C: An acid increases the concentration of H^+ ions when it is dissolved in water. It is a proton donor in a chemical equation, or acts an electron-pair acceptor. A base increases the concentration of OH^- ions when it is dissolved in water, accepts a proton in a chemical reaction, or is an electron-pair donor. Therefore, only Choice C is correct.

21. A: A synthesis reaction occurs when two or more elements or compounds are joined together to form a single product. Choice A shows the chemical equation for the synthesis of nitrogen dioxide (NO_2) from nitric oxide (NO) and oxygen (O_2). Choice B is a decomposition reaction because a single reactant (carbonic acid, which is in soft drinks) is broken down into two or more products (in this case, water and carbon dioxide). Choices C and D are single displacement reactions, which occur when a single element or ion takes the place of another element in a compound.

22. B: The reaction between methane (CH_4) and oxygen is a combustion reaction, which is a special type of double displacement reaction. Double displacement reactions occur when two elements or ions exchange a single element to form two different compounds. This means that the final compounds have different combinations of cations and anions than the reactants did. Redox reactions and acid-base reactions are also special types of double replacement reactions. In combustion reactions, a hydrocarbon reacts with oxygen to form carbon dioxide and water.

23. B: The percent yield for a reaction is the actual yield is divided by the theoretical yield and then multiplied by 100. Since 65 grams of CaO were expected, this value is the theoretical yield. The actual yield is the 45 grams produced. Thus, the percent yield is: $\frac{45\ grams}{65\ grams} \times 100 = \times 69\%$.

24. B: An atom, ion, or molecule that loses electrons and becomes more positively charged has been oxidized. A substance is reduced when it gains electrons and becomes more negatively charged. Choices C and D are incorrect because when electrons, which carry a negative charge are lost, the amount of negative charge of the substance that lost them becomes less. Therefore, the charge of the substance that lost the electrons becomes less negative or more positive.

25. A: A conjugate base is the ion that is formed when an acid it is paired with loses a proton. HSO_4^- is the conjugate base of the acid H_2SO_4. Choice B is incorrect because it reverses the relationship. Remember that the acid donates a proton, so the conjugate base pair of an acid has the same molecular formula of the acid, except it has one fewer proton (H^+). Therefore, the conjugate base ion has lost a positive charge, so it should have a negative charge. Thus, Choice C is incorrect.

Anatomy and Physiology

1. A: The cells of connective tissue are dispersed throughout a gelatinous, liquid, protein fiber, or mineral salt matrix. Retinaculum is one of the primary protein fibers in the matrix, along with collagen (for strength) and elastin (for flexibility). It mainly provides support and is one of the primary constituents in retinacular connective tissue, which helps support structures such as lymph organs.

2. B: The innermost epidermal tissue is a single layer of cells called the stratum basale. The melanocytes in the stratum basale produce melanin, an important pigment that absorbs UV rays to protect the skin from sun damage. The outermost epidermal layer, called the stratum corneum, helps repel water; therefore, Choice A is incorrect. The stratum granulosum produces keratin, so Choice C is incorrect. The dermis, which is underneath the epidermis, contains the oil glands that produce and secrete oil.

3. D: Veins have valves, but arteries do not. Valves in veins are designed to prevent backflow, since they are the furthest blood vessels from the pumping action of the heart and steadily increase in volume (which decreases the available pressure). Capillaries diffuse nutrients properly because of their thin walls and high surface area and are not particularly dependent on positive pressure.

4. D: Cartilage is avascular, which is one reason why it is limited in its ability to repair itself following an injury. It receives materials such as nutrients via diffusion.

5. D: The smallest functional unit of the body is the cell. Groups of similar cells are arranged into *tissues,* such as nervous tissue, epithelial tissue, and adipose tissue. From there, different tissues are arranged into *organs,* and organs that work together form entire *organ systems.*

6. C: Oil glands, like sweat glands, are exocrine glands of the skin. Oil glands, which are attached to hair follicles, secrete sebum. Sebum is an oily substance that moisturizes the skin, protects it from water loss, helps keep the skin elastic, and provides a chemical defense against bacterial and fungal infections due to its slight acidity. Evaporative cooling, which is when the hottest water particles on the skin evaporate and leave behind the coolest ones to help cool the body, is not a function of sebum. In hot conditions, the hypothalamus will initiate a pathway that vasodilates blood vessels near the surface of the skin to increase heat loss and stimulate sweating.

7. A: Skeletal muscle fibers are made of myofibrils, which interact when a muscle contracts in a model called the sliding filament theory. The myofibrils are arranged in each muscle fibers in functional units called sarcomeres. The thicker filaments, called myosin, are in between the thinner actin filaments, which are anchored to Z lines. One sarcomere is defined as the region between two adjacent Z lines.

Myosin filaments are attached to a central M line. When a muscle is at rest, there is a gap between the Z line and the myosin filaments; in fact, it is the arrangement of filaments that gives skeletal muscle its striated appearance. When the muscle contracts, the heads of the myosin filaments attach to the actin and form cross-bridges, which are used to pull the actin filaments closer to the M line.

8. D: Epithelial tissue covers the external surfaces of organs and lines many of the body's cavities. It can be arranged into four patterns. Transitional epithelium is noted for its ability to expand and contract. Choice A is incorrect because it describes simple epithelial tissue. Choice B is incorrect because it describes pseudostratified epithelial tissue. Choice C is incorrect because although transitional epithelial tissue does help protect the body from invading microbes, this ability is not unique to transitional epithelium. Instead, it is a shared characteristic of all epithelial tissue.

9. A: Antibodies. Antibiotics (B) fight bacteria, but the body does not make them naturally. White blood cells, not red blood cells (D) are the blood cells produced that fight the bacteria. Vaccines (C) are given to create antibodies and prevent future illness.

10. B: Red blood cells are the chief transport vehicle for oxygen. Red blood cells contain hemoglobin, a protein that helps transport oxygen throughout the circulatory system.

11. A: Choice B might be an attractive answer choice, but neutrophils are part of the innate immune system and are not considered part of the primary immune response. The first event that happens in a primary immune response is that macrophages ingest pathogens and display their antigens. Then, they secrete interleukin 1 to recruit helper T cells. Once helper T cells are activated, they secrete interleukin 2 to simulate plasma B and killer T cell production. Only then can plasma B make the pathogen specific antibodies.

12. C: The epididymis stores sperm and is a coiled tube located near the testes. The immature sperm that enters the epididymis from the testes migrates through the 20-foot long epididymis tube in about two weeks, where viable sperm are concentrated at the end. The vas deferens is a tube that transports mature sperm from the epididymis to the urethra. Seminal vesicles are pouches attached that add fructose to the ejaculate to provide energy for sperm. The prostate gland excretes fluid that makes up about a third of semen released during ejaculation. The fluid reduces semen viscosity and contains enzymes that aid in sperm functioning; both effects increase sperm motility and ultimate success.

13. C: The female reproductive system is a symphony of different hormones that work together in order to propagate the species. Below, find the function of each one:

Hormone	Source	Action
GnRH	Hypothalamus	Stimulates anterior pituitary to secrete FSH and LH
FSH	Anterior Pituitary	Stimulates ovaries to develop mature follicles (with ova); follicles produce increasingly high levels of estrogen
LH	Anterior Pituitary	Stimulates the release of the ovum by the follicle; follicle then converted into a corpus luteum that secretes progesterone
Estrogen	Ovary (follicle); placenta	Stimulates repair of endometrium of uterus; negative feedback effect inhibits hypothalamus production of GnRH
Progesterone	Ovary (corpus luteum); placenta	Stimulates thickening of and maintains endometrium; negative feedback inhibits pituitary production of LH
Prolactin	Anterior pituitary	Stimulates milk production after childbirth
Oxytocin	Posterior pituitary	Stimulates milk "letdown"
Androgens	Adrenal glands	Stimulates sexual drive
hCG	Embryo (if pregnancy)	Stimulates production of progesterone

14. A: Epithelial cells line cavities and surfaces of body organs and glands, and the three main shapes are squamous, columnar, and cuboidal. Epithelial cells contain no blood vessels, and their functions involve absorption, protection, transport, secretion, and sensing. Simple squamous epithelial are flat cells that are present in lungs and line the heart and vessels. Their flat shape aids in their function, which is diffusion of materials. Simple cuboidal epithelium is found in ducts, and simple columnar epithelium is found in tubes with projections (uterus, villi, bronchi). Any of these types of epithelial cells can be stacked, and then they are called stratified and not simple.

15. B: The position of the clavicle relative to the humerus is medial. Anatomical directions are referenced to the midline (medial, and lateral); to the center (proximal and distal); to the front and rear (anterior and posterior); toward the head and tail (cephalic and caudal); and to the head and feet (superior and inferior). In anatomical position, the body stands erect with palms facing forward. The clavicle would be clearly medial and superior to the humerus as it is closer to the midline and head.

16. A: The coronal, or frontal, plane is a vertical plane positioned so that it divides the body into front (ventral) and back (dorsal) regions. The plane is positioned so that the face, kneecap, and toes are on the ventral side, and the vertebrae and heel are on the dorsal side. The coronal plane is one of three body planes. The other two are the transverse and sagittal planes. The transverse plane divides the anatomy into upper (cranial or head) and lower (caudal or tail) regions. The sagittal plane runs front/back perpendicular to the frontal plane and divides the anatomy into right and left regions.

17. C: Cartilage adds mechanical support to joints. It provides a flexible cushion that aids in mobility while offering support. The first two choices are switched—it is ligaments that connect bones at joints and tendons that attach skeletal muscles to bones. *D* is incorrect because arteries, not veins, deliver oxygenated blood.

18. B: The dermis is the skin layer that contains nerves, blood vessels, hair follicles, and glands. These structures are called skin appendages. These appendages are scattered throughout the connective tissue (elastin and collagen), and the connective tissue provides support to the outer layer, the epidermis. The epidermal surface is a thin layer (except feet and palms where it is thick) of continually-regenerating cells that don't have a blood supply of their own, which explains why superficial cuts don't bleed. The hypodermis is the subcutaneous layer underneath the dermis, and it is composed primary of fat in order to provide insulation.

19. D: Receptors in the dermis help the body maintain homeostasis, for example, in terms of regulating body temperature. Signals travel to the hypothalamus, which then secretes hormones that activate effectors to keep internal temperature at a set point of 98.6°F (37°C). For example, if the environment is too cold, the hypothalamus will initiate a pathway that will cause the muscles to shiver because shivering helps heat the body.

20. B: The radius and ulna are the bones from the elbow to the wrist, and the humerus is the bone between the elbow and the shoulder. The tibia and fibula are the bones from the knee to the ankle, and the femur is the bone from the knee to the hip. The other choices are bones in the body as well, just not limb bones. The mandible is the jaw, the scapula is the shoulder blade, and the carpal bones are in the wrist.

21. B: In the Haversian system found in compact bone, concentric layers of bone cells are called lamellae. Between the lamellae are lacunae, which are gaps filled with osteocytes. The Haversian canals on the outer regions of the bone contain capillaries and nerve fibers. Spongy (cancellous) bone is on the extremities of long bones, which makes sense because the ends are softer due to the motion at joints (providing flexibility and cushion). The middle of the bone between the two spongy regions is called the diaphysis region. Spongy bone is highly vascular and is the site of red bone marrow (the marrow that makes red blood cells). Long bones, on the other hand, are long, weight-bearing bones like the tibia or femur that contain yellow marrow in adulthood. Trabeculae is a dense, collagenous, rod-shaped tissue that add mechanical support to the spongy regions of bone. Muscular trabeculae can be found in the heart and are similar in that the offer physical reinforcement.

22. A: Carbon dioxide rich blood is delivered and collected in the right atrium and moved to the right ventricle. The tricuspid valve prevents backflow between the two chambers. From there, the pulmonary artery takes blood to the lungs where diffusion causes gas exchange. Then, blood collects in the left atrium and moves to the left ventricle. The mitral valve prevents the backflow of blood from the ventricle to the atrium. Finally, blood is pumped to the body and released in the aorta.

23. B: Smooth, skeletal, and cardiac muscle have defining characteristics, due to their vastly different functions. All have actin and myosin microfilaments that slide past each other to contract.

Skeletal muscles have long fibers made of clearly defined sarcomeres, which make them appear striated. Sarcomeres consist of alternating dark A bands (thick myosin) and light I bands (thin actin). Upon muscle contraction, fibers slide past each. Skeletal muscles are attached to bone via tendons and are responsible for voluntary movement; their contraction brings bones together. They contain multiple nuclei, due to their bundling into fibers.

Cardiac muscles also contain sarcomeres and appear striated, but are branched cells with a single nucleus. Branching allows each cell to connect with several others, forming a huge network that has more strength (the whole is greater than the sum of its parts).

Smooth muscles are non-striated and are responsible for involuntary movement (digestion). They do not form cylindrical fibers like skeletal muscles. Their lack of striations is because they have no sarcomeres, and the filaments are randomly arranged.

24. B: The reflex arc is the simplest nerve pathway. The stimulus bypasses the brain, going from sensory receptors through an afferent (incoming) neuron to the spinal cord. It synapses with an efferent (outgoing) neuron in the spinal cord and is transmitted directly to muscle. There is no interneuron involved in a reflex arc. The classic example of a reflex arc is the knee jerk response. Tapping on the patellar tendon of the knee stretches the quadriceps muscle of the thigh, resulting in contraction of the muscle and extension of the knee.

25. D: Bony matrix is an intricate lattice of collagen fibers and mineral salts, particularly calcium and phosphorus. The mineral salts are strong but brittle, and the collagen fibers are weak but flexible, so the combination of the two makes bone resistant to shattering and able to withstand the normal forces applied to it.

Physics

1. B: Convection is the transfer of heat due to the movement of molecules from an area of higher concentration to that of lower concentration; this is also how heat can travel throughout a house to warm each room. Conduction is the transfer of energy from one molecule to another molecule through actually touching or making contact with each other. Radiation is how the sun warms the earth; no medium is needed for this type of transfer.

2. C: When conducting scientific research, it is best to rely on sources that are known for honest, ethical, and unbiased research and experimentation. Most laboratories and universities must have their work validated through independent means in order to publish or claim results. Anyone can publish things on the Internet—it does not mean their work has been validated, and therefore, their work may not be correct.

3. D: Sublimation is a change in state from a solid to a gas. Evaporation is a change in state from a liquid to a gas, melting is a change in state from a solid to a liquid, and condensation is a change in state from a gas to a liquid.

4. D: Mass refers to the amount or quantity there is of an object. Light, sound, and heat are all forms of energy that can travel in waves.

5. A: The mechanical energy is the total (or sum) of the potential energy and the kinetic energy at any given point in a system.

$$ME = PE + KE; 50\ Joules = 30\ Joules + 20\ Joules$$

6. B: It appears to bend because of the refraction of light traveling from air to water. When light travels from one material to another it can reflect, refract, and go through different materials. Choice *A* is incorrect, as the pencil does not actually become warped but only *appears* to be warped. Choice *C* is incorrect; although the pencil appears to bend because of its immersion into separate mediums where speed is different, the pencil does not become temporarily warped—it only appears to be warped. Choice *D* is incorrect; it is the refraction of light, not reflection. The latter happens within the same medium, which makes the answer choice incorrect.

7. A: According to Ohm's Law: *V* = *IR*, so using the given variables: 3.0 V = I × 6.0 Ω

Solving for I: I = 3.0 V/6.0 Ω = 0.5 A

Choice *B* incorporates a miscalculation in the equation by multiplying 3.0 V by 6.0 Ω, rather than dividing these values. Choices *C* and *D* are labeled with the wrong units; Joules measure energy, not current.

8. C: This is a fundamental law of thermodynamics. Energy can only transfer, transform, or travel. The amount of energy in a system is always the same.

9. D: When electricity is run through a wire, it is carrying current and current has a charge. Therefore, there is a charge running down the wire, which creates a magnetic field that can attract and repel just like any magnet.

10. C: In any system, the total mechanical energy is the sum of the potential energy and the kinetic energy. Either value could be zero but it still must be included in the total. Choices *A* and *B* only give the total potential or kinetic energy, respectively. Choice *D* gives the difference in the kinetic and potential energy.

HESI A2 Practice Test #2

Mathematics

1. If a car can travel 300 miles in 4 hours, how far can it go in an hour and a half?
    a. 100 miles
    b. 112.5 miles
    c. 135.5 miles
    d. 150 miles

2. At the store, Jan spends $90 on apples and oranges. Apples cost $1 each and oranges cost $2 each. If Jan buys the same number of apples as oranges, how many oranges did she buy?
    a. 20
    b. 25
    c. 30
    d. 35

3. What is the volume of a box with rectangular sides 5 feet long, 6 feet wide, and 3 feet high?
    a. 60 cubic feet
    b. 75 cubic feet
    c. 90 cubic feet
    d. 14 cubic feet

4. A train traveling 50 miles per hour takes a trip lasting 3 hours. If a map has a scale of 1 inch per 10 miles, how many inches apart are the train's starting point and ending point on the map?
    a. 14
    b. 12
    c. 13
    d. 15

5. A traveler takes an hour to drive to a museum, spends 3 hours and 30 minutes there, and takes half an hour to drive home. What percentage of his or her time was spent driving?
    a. 15%
    b. 30%
    c. 40%
    d. 60%

6. A truck is carrying three cylindrical barrels. Their bases have a diameter of 2 feet and they have a height of 3 feet. What is the total volume of all three barrels in cubic feet?
    a. 3π
    b. 9π
    c. 12π
    d. 15π

7. Greg buys a $10 lunch with 5% sales tax. He leaves a $2 tip after his bill. How much money does he spend?
    a. $12.50
    b. $12
    c. $13
    d. $13.25

8. Marty wishes to save $150 over a 4-day period. How much must Marty save each day on average?
    a. $37.50
    b. $35
    c. $45.50
    d. $41

9. Bernard can make $80 per day. If he needs to make $300 and only works full days, how many days will this take?
    a. 6
    b. 3
    c. 5
    d. 4

10. A couple buys a house for $150,000. They sell it for $165,000. By what percentage did the house's value increase?
    a. 10%
    b. 13%
    c. 15%
    d. 17%

11. A school has 15 teachers and 20 teaching assistants. They have 200 students. What is the ratio of faculty to students?
    a. 3:20
    b. 4:17
    c. 5:54
    d. 7:40

12. A map has a scale of 1 inch per 5 miles. A car can travel 60 miles per hour. If the distance from the start to the destination is 3 inches on the map, how long will it take the car to make the trip?
    a. 12 minutes
    b. 15 minutes
    c. 17 minutes
    d. 20 minutes

13. Taylor works two jobs. The first pays $20,000 per year. The second pays $10,000 per year. She donates 15% of her income to charity. How much does she donate each year?
    a. $4500
    b. $5000
    c. $5500
    d. $6000

14. A box with rectangular sides is 24 inches wide, 18 inches deep, and 12 inches high. What is the volume of the box in cubic feet?

    a. 2

    b. 3

    c. 4

    d. 5

15. Kristen purchases $100 worth of CDs and DVDs. The CDs cost $10 each and the DVDs cost $15. If she bought four DVDs, how many CDs did she buy?

    a. 5

    b. 6

    c. 3

    d. 4

16. If Sarah reads at an average rate of 21 pages in four nights, how long will it take her to read 140 pages?

    a. 6 nights

    b. 26 nights

    c. 8 nights

    d. 27 nights

17. Mom's car drove 72 miles in 90 minutes. There are 5280 feet per mile. How fast did she drive in feet per second?

    a. 0.8 feet per second

    b. 48.9 feet per second

    c. 0.009 feet per second

    d. 70. 4 feet per second

18. This chart indicates how many sales of CDs, vinyl records, and MP3 downloads occurred over the last year. Approximately what percentage of the total sales was from CDs?

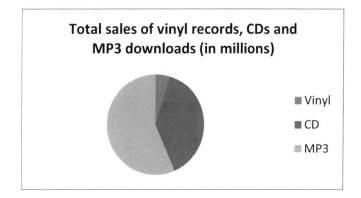

    a. 55%

    b. 25%

    c. 40%

    d. 5%

19. After a 20% sale discount, Frank purchased a new refrigerator for $850. How much did he save from the original price?
    a. $170
    b. $212.50
    c. $105.75
    d. $200

20. 3.4+2.35+4=
    a. 5.35
    b. 9.2
    c. 9.75
    d. 10.25

21. $5.88 \times 3.2 =$
    a. 18.816
    b. 16.44
    c. 20.352
    d. 17

22. $\frac{3}{25} =$
    a. 0.15
    b. 0.1
    c. 0.9
    d. 0.12

23. Which of the following is largest?
    a. 0.45
    b. 0.096
    c. 0.3
    d. 0.313

24. Which of the following is NOT a way to write 40 percent of N?
    a. $(0.4)N$
    b. $\frac{2}{5}N$
    c. $40N$
    d. $\frac{4N}{10}$

25. Which is closest to 17.8×9.9?
    a. 140
    b. 180
    c. 200
    d. 350

26. A student gets an 85% on a test with 20 questions. How many answers did the student solve correctly?

    a. 15

    b. 16

    c. 17

    d. 18

27. Four people split a bill. The first person pays for $\frac{1}{5}$, the second person pays for $\frac{1}{4}$, and the third person pays for $\frac{1}{3}$. What fraction of the bill does the fourth person pay?

    a. $\frac{13}{60}$

    b. $\frac{47}{60}$

    c. $\frac{1}{4}$

    d. $\frac{4}{15}$

28. 6 is 30% of what number?

    a. 18

    b. 20

    c. 24

    d. 26

29. $2\frac{1}{3} - 2\frac{1}{5} =$

    a. $\frac{2}{15}$

    b. $\frac{1}{15}$

    c. $\frac{1}{3}$

    d. $\frac{1}{5}$

30. What is $\frac{420}{98}$ rounded to the nearest integer?

    a. 4

    b. 3

    c. 5

    d. 6

31. $4\frac{1}{3} + 3\frac{3}{4} =$

    a. $6\frac{5}{12}$

    b. $8\frac{1}{12}$

    c. $8\frac{2}{3}$

    d. $7\frac{7}{12}$

32. Five of six numbers have a sum of 25. The average of all six numbers is 6. What is the sixth number?

    a. 8

    b. 10

    c. 11

    d. 12

33. $52.3 \times 10^{-3} =$
    a. 0.00523
    b. 0.0523
    c. 0.523
    d. 523

34. If $\frac{5}{2} \div \frac{1}{3} = n$, then n is between:
    a. 5 and 7
    b. 7 and 9
    c. 9 and 11
    d. 3 and 5

35. A closet is filled with red, blue, and green shirts. If $\frac{1}{3}$ of the shirts are green and $\frac{2}{5}$ are red, what fraction of the shirts are blue?
    a. $\frac{4}{15}$
    b. $\frac{1}{5}$
    c. $\frac{7}{15}$
    d. $\frac{1}{2}$

36. Shawna buys $2\frac{1}{2}$ gallons of paint. If she uses $\frac{1}{3}$ of it on the first day, how much does she have left?
    a. $1\frac{5}{6}$ gallons
    b. $1\frac{1}{2}$ gallons
    c. $1\frac{2}{3}$ gallons
    d. 2 gallons

37. A drug needs to be stored at room temperature (68 °F). What is the equivalent temperature in degrees Celsius?
    a. 36 °C
    b. 72 °C
    c. 68 °C
    d. 20 °C

38. Add $4.33 + 7.688$.
    a. 12.018
    b. 3.358
    c. 8.121
    d. 33.289

39. Add and express in reduced form $7/12 + 2/9$.
    a. 9/12
    b. 14/108
    c. 29/36
    d. 2/3

40. Subtract 37.517 − 18.664.
   a. 18.853
   b. 56.181
   c. 35.6506
   d. 18.032

41. Subtract 401.2 − 82.56.
   a. 118.66
   b. 318.64
   c. 315.94
   d. 483.76

42. Subtract and express in reduced form 39/45 − 8/15.
   a. 15/45
   b. 31/45
   c. 2/3
   d. 1/3

43. Multiply 13.7 × 0.3.
   a. 45.66
   b. 4.11
   c. 14.0
   d. 41.1

44. Multiply 1,413 × 0.07.
   a. 1414
   b. 98.91
   c. 989.1
   d. 9.891

45. Multiply and reduce 15/21 × 48/108.
   a. 20/63
   b. 33/87
   c. 60/189
   d. 720/2268

46. Divide, express with a fraction remainder 1,107 ÷ 34.
   a. 31 39/34
   b. 3 29/34
   c. 32/34
   d. 32 19/34

47. Divide and reduce 14/28 ÷ 23/9.
   a. 9/19
   b. 9/23
   c. 9/46
   d. 23/46

48. Express as a reduced mixed number 55/12.
    a. 4 7/12
    b. 4 7/55
    c. 4 3/12
    d. 4 12/55

49. Express as an improper fraction 9 5/6.
    a. 54/6
    b. 59/6
    c. 45/6
    d. 45/9

50. Round to the nearest thousandth 2,718.0354.
    a. 3,000
    b. 2,718.04
    c. 2,718.035
    d. 2,718.036

Reading Comprehension

Questions 1–3 are based on the following poem:

The Old Man and His Grandson

There was once a very old man, whose eyes had become dim,

his ears dull of hearing, his knees trembled, and when he sat at

table he could hardly hold the spoon, and spilt the broth upon

the table-cloth or let it run out of his mouth. His son and his

son's wife were disgusted at this, so the old grandfather at last

had to sit in the corner behind the stove, and they gave him his

food in an earthenware bowl, and not even enough of it. And he

used to look towards the table with his eyes full of tears. Once,

too, his trembling hands could not hold the bowl, and it fell to

the ground and broke. The young wife scolded him, but he said

nothing and only sighed. Then they brought him a wooden

bowl for a few half-pence, out of which he had to eat.

They were once sitting thus when the little grandson of four

years old began to gather together some bits of wood upon the ground. 'What are you doing there?' asked the father. 'I am making a little trough,' answered the child, 'for father and mother to eat out of when I am big.'

The man and his wife looked at each other for a while, and presently began to cry. Then they took the old grandfather to the table, and henceforth always let him eat with them, and likewise said nothing if he did spill a little of anything.

(Grimms' Fairy Tales, p. 111)

1. Which of the following most accurately represents the theme of the passage?
   a. Respect your elders
   b. Children will follow their parents' example
   c. You reap what you sow
   d. Loyalty will save your life

2. Which character trait most accurately reflects the son and his wife in this story?
   a. Compassion
   b. Understanding
   c. Cruelty
   d. Impatience

3. Why do the son and his wife decide to let the old man sit at the table?
   a. Because they felt sorry for him
   b. Because their son told them to
   c. Because the old man would not stop crying
   d. Because they saw their own actions in their son

Questions 4–9 are based on the following excerpt from a novel set in nineteenth-century France, where two friends, Albert de Morcef and the Count of Monte Cristo, discuss Parisian social life.

"Mademoiselle Eugénie is pretty—I think I remember that to be her name."

"Very pretty, or rather, very beautiful," replied Albert, "but of that style of beauty which I don't appreciate; I am an ungrateful fellow."

"Really," said Monte Cristo, lowering his voice, "you don't appear to me to be very enthusiastic on the subject of this marriage."

"Mademoiselle Danglars is too rich for me," replied Morcerf, "and that frightens me."

"Bah," exclaimed Monte Cristo, "that's a fine reason to give. Are you not rich yourself?"

"My father's income is about 50,000 francs per annum; and he will give me, perhaps, ten or twelve thousand when I marry."

"That, perhaps, might not be considered a large sum, in Paris especially," said the count; "but everything doesn't depend on wealth, and it's a fine thing to have a good name, and to occupy a high station in society. Your name is celebrated, your position magnificent; and then the Comte de Morcerf is a soldier, and it's pleasing to see the integrity of a Bayard united to the poverty of a Duguesclin; disinterestedness is the brightest ray in which a noble sword can shine. As for me, I consider the union with Mademoiselle Danglars a most suitable one; she will enrich you, and you will ennoble her."

Albert shook his head, and looked thoughtful. "There is still something else," said he.

"I confess," observed Monte Cristo, "that I have some difficulty in comprehending your objection to a young lady who is both rich and beautiful."

"Oh," said Morcerf, "this repugnance, if repugnance it may be called, isn't all on my side."

"Whence can it arise, then? for you told me your father desired the marriage."

"It's my mother who dissents; she has a clear and penetrating judgment, and doesn't smile on the proposed union. I cannot account for it, but she seems to entertain some prejudice against the Danglars."

"Ah," said the count, in a somewhat forced tone, "that may be easily explained; the Comtesse de Morcerf, who is aristocracy and refinement itself, doesn't relish the idea of being allied by your marriage with one of ignoble birth; that is natural enough."

4. What can be inferred about Albert's family?
   a. Their finances are uncertain.
   b. Albert is the only son in his family.
   c. Their name is more respected than the Danglars'.
   d. Albert's mother and father both agree on their decisions.

5. What is Albert's attitude towards his impending marriage?
   a. Pragmatic
   b. Romantic
   c. Indifferent
   d. Apprehensive

6. What is the best description of the Count's relationship with Albert?
   a. He's like a strict parent, criticizing Albert's choices.
   b. He's like a wise uncle, giving practical advice to Albert.
   c. He's like a close friend, supporting all of Albert's opinions.
   d. He's like a suspicious investigator, asking many probing questions.

7. Which sentence is true of Albert's mother?
   a. She belongs to a noble family.
   b. She often makes poor choices.
   c. She is primarily occupied with money.
   d. She is unconcerned about her son's future.

8. Based on this passage, what is probably NOT true about French society in the 1800s?
   a. Children often received money from their parents.
   b. Marriages were sometimes arranged between families.
   c. The richest people in society were also the most respected.
   d. People were often expected to marry within their same social class.

9. Why is the Count puzzled by Albert's attitude toward his marriage?
   a. He seems reluctant to marry Eugénie, despite her wealth and beauty.
   b. He is marrying against his father's wishes, despite usually following his advice.
   c. He appears excited to marry someone he doesn't love, despite being a hopeless romantic.
   d. He expresses reverence towards Eugénie, despite being from a higher social class than her.

Questions 10-18 are based upon the following passage:

The Global Water Crisis

For decades, the world's water supply has been decreasing. At least ten percent of the world population, or over 780 million people, do not have access to potable water. They have to walk for miles, carrying heavy buckets in intense heat in order to obtain the essential life source that comes freely from our faucets.

We are in a global water crisis. Only 2.5% of the water on Earth is suitable for drinking, and over seventy percent of this water is frozen in the polar ice caps, while much of the rest is located deep underground. This leaves a very small percentage available for drinking, yet we see millions of gallons of water wasted on watering huge lawns in deserts like Arizona, or on running dishwashers that are only half-full, or on filling all the personal pools in Los Angeles, meanwhile people in Africa are dying of thirst.

In order to reduce water waste, Americans and citizens of other first world countries should adhere to the following guidelines: run the dishwasher only when it is full, do only full loads of laundry, wash the car with a bucket and not with a hose, take showers only when necessary, swim in public pools, and just be cognizant of how much water they are using in general. Our planet is getting thirstier by the year, and if we do not solve this problem, our species will surely perish.

10. Which of the following best supports the assertion that we need to limit our water usage?
    a. People are wasting water on superfluous things.
    b. There is very little water on earth suitable for drinking.
    c. At least ten percent of the world population does not have access to drinking water.
    d. There is plenty of drinking water in first world countries, but not anywhere else.

11. How is the content in the selection organized?
    a. In chronological order
    b. Compare and contrast
    c. As a set of problems and solutions
    d. As a series of descriptions

12. The passage is told from what point of view?
    a. First person
    b. Second person
    c. Third person
    d. Both A and B

13. Which of the following, if true, would challenge the assertion that we are in a global water crisis?
    a. There are abundant water stores on earth that scientists are not reporting.
    b. Much of the water we drink comes from rain.
    c. People in Africa only have to walk less than a mile to get water.
    d. Most Americans only run the dishwasher when it is full.

14. The selection is written in which of the following styles?
    a. As a narrative
    b. In a persuasive manner
    c. As an informative piece
    d. As a series of descriptions

15. Which of the following is implicitly stated within the following sentence? "This leaves a very small percentage available for drinking, yet we see millions of gallons of water wasted on watering huge lawns in deserts like Arizona, or on running dishwashers that are only half-full, or on filling all the personal pools in Los Angeles, meanwhile people in Africa are dying of thirst."
    a. People run dishwashers that are not full.
    b. People in Africa are dying of thirst.
    c. People take water for granted.
    d. People should stop watering their lawns.

16. Why does the author mention that people have to walk for miles in intense heat to get water?
    a. To inform the reader on the hardships of living in a third world country.
    b. To inspire compassion in the reader.
    c. To show that water is only available in first world countries.
    d. To persuade the reader to reduce their water usage.

17. What is meant by the word <u>cognizant</u>?
    a. To be interested
    b. To be amused
    c. To be mindful
    d. To be accepting

18. What is the main idea of the passage?
    a. People should reduce their water usage.
    b. There is very little drinking water on earth.
    c. People take their access to water for granted.
    d. People should swim in public pools.

Questions 19–21 refer to the following paragraph:

The Brookside area is an older part of Kansas City, developed mainly in the 1920s and 30s, and is considered one of the nation's first "planned" communities with shops, restaurants, parks, and churches all within a quick walk. A stroll down any street reveals charming two-story Tudor and Colonial homes with smaller bungalows sprinkled throughout the beautiful tree-lined streets. It is common to see lemonade stands on the corners and baseball games in the numerous "pocket" parks tucked neatly behind rows of well-manicured houses. The Brookside shops on 63rd street between Wornall Road and Oak Street are a hub of commerce and entertainment where residents freely shop and dine with their pets (and children) in tow. This is also a common "hangout" spot for younger teenagers because it is easily accessible by bike for most. In short, it is an idyllic neighborhood just minutes from downtown Kansas City.

19. Which of the following states the main idea of this paragraph?
    a. The Brookside shops are a popular hangout for teenagers.
    b. There are a number of pocket parks in the Brookside neighborhood.
    c. Brookside is a great place to live.
    d. Brookside has a high crime rate.

20. In what kind of publication might you read the above paragraph?
    a. Fictional novel
    b. Community profile
    c. Newspaper article
    d. Movie review

21. According to this paragraph, which of the following is unique to this neighborhood?
    a. It is old.
    b. It is in Kansas City.
    c. It has shopping.
    d. It is one of the nation's first planned communities.

Questions 22–25 refer to the following passage, titled "Education is Essential to Civilization."

Early in my career, a master teacher shared this thought with me: "Education is the last bastion of civility." While I did not completely understand the scope of those words at the time, I have since come to realize the depth, breadth, truth, and significance of what he said. Education provides society with a vehicle for raising its children to be civil, decent, human beings with something valuable to contribute to the world. It is really what makes us human and what distinguishes us as civilized creatures.

Being "civilized" humans means being "whole" humans. Education must address the mind, body, and soul of students. It would be detrimental to society if our schools were myopic in their focus, only meeting the needs of the mind. As humans, we are multi-dimensional, multi-faceted beings who need more than head knowledge to survive. The human heart and psyche have to be fed in order for the mind to develop properly, and the body must be maintained and exercised to help fuel the working of the brain.

Education is a basic human right, and it allows us to sustain a democratic society in which participation is fundamental to its success. It should inspire students to seek better solutions to world problems and to dream of a more equitable society. Education should never discriminate on any basis, and it should create individuals who are self-sufficient, patriotic, and tolerant of other's ideas.

All children can learn, although not all children learn in the same manner. All children learn best, however, when their basic physical needs are met, and they feel safe, secure, and loved. Students are much more responsive to a teacher who values them and shows them respect as individual people. Teachers must model at all times the way they expect students to treat them and their peers. If teachers set high expectations for their students, the students will rise to that high level. Teachers must make the well-being of their students their primary focus and must not be afraid to let their students learn from their own mistakes.

In the modern age of technology, a teacher's focus is no longer the "what" of the content, but more importantly, the "why." Students are bombarded with information and have access to ANY information they need right at their fingertips. Teachers have to work harder than ever before to help students identify salient information and to think critically about the information they encounter. Students have to read between the lines, identify bias, and determine who they can trust in the milieu of ads, data, and texts presented to them.

Schools must work in consort with families in this important mission. While children spend most of their time in school, they are dramatically and indelibly shaped by the influences of their family and culture. Teachers must not only respect this fact but must strive to include parents in the education of their children and must work to keep parents informed of progress and problems. Communication between classroom and home is essential for a child's success.

Humans have always aspired to be more, do more, and to better ourselves and our communities. This is where education lies, right at the heart of humanity's desire to be all that we can be. Education helps us strive for higher goals and better treatment of ourselves and others. I shudder to think what would become of us if education ceased to be the "last bastion of civility." We must be unapologetic about expecting excellence from our students—our very existence depends upon it.

22. Which of the following best summarizes the author's main point?
    a. Education as we know it is over-valued in modern society, and we should find alternative solutions.
    b. The survival of the human race depends on the educational system, and it is worth fighting for to make it better.
    c. The government should do away with all public schools and require parents to home school their children instead.
    d. While education is important, some children simply are not capable of succeeding in a traditional classroom.

23. Based on this passage, which of the following can be inferred about the author?
    a. The author feels passionately about education.
    b. The author does not feel strongly about his point.
    c. The author is angry at the educational system.
    d. The author is unsure about the importance of education.

24. Based on this passage, which of the following conclusions could be drawn about the author?
    a. The author would not support raising taxes to help fund much needed reforms in education.
    b. The author would support raising taxes to help fund much needed reforms in education, as long as those reforms were implemented in higher socio-economic areas first.
    c. The author would support raising taxes to help fund much needed reforms in education for all children in all schools.
    d. The author would support raising taxes only in certain states to help fund much needed reforms in education.

25. According to the passage, which of the following is not mentioned as an important factor in education today?

    a. Parent involvement

    b. Communication between parents and teachers

    c. Impact of technology

    d. Cost of textbooks

Questions 26–28 are based upon the following passage:

This excerpt is adaptation from Charles Dickens' speech in Birmingham in England on December 30, 1853 on behalf of the Birmingham and Midland Institute.

My Good Friends,—When I first imparted to the committee of the projected Institute my particular wish that on one of the evenings of my readings here the main body of my audience should be composed of working men and their families, I was animated by two desires; first, by the wish to have the great pleasure of meeting you face to face at this Christmas time, and accompany you myself through one of my little Christmas books; and second, by the wish to have an opportunity of stating publicly in your presence, and in the presence of the committee, my earnest hope that the Institute will, from the beginning, recognise one great principle—strong in reason and justice—which I believe to be essential to the very life of such an Institution. It is, that the working man shall, from the first unto the last, have a share in the management of an Institution which is designed for his benefit, and which calls itself by his name.

I have no fear here of being misunderstood—of being supposed to mean too much in this. If there ever was a time when any one class could of itself do much for its own good, and for the welfare of society—which I greatly doubt—that time is unquestionably past. It is in the fusion of different classes, without confusion; in the bringing together of employers and employed; in the creating of a better common understanding among those whose interests are identical, who depend upon each other, who are vitally essential to each other, and who never can be in unnatural antagonism without deplorable results, that one of the chief principles of a Mechanics' Institution should consist. In this world a great deal of the bitterness among us arises from an imperfect understanding of one another. Erect in Birmingham a great Educational Institution, properly educational; educational of the feelings as well as of the reason; to which all orders of Birmingham men contribute; in which all orders of Birmingham men meet; wherein all orders of Birmingham men are faithfully represented—and you will erect a Temple of Concord here which will be a model edifice to the whole of England.

Contemplating as I do the existence of the Artisans' Committee, which not long ago considered the establishment of the Institute so sensibly, and supported it so heartily, I earnestly entreat the gentlemen—earnest I know in the good work, and who are now among us,—by all means to avoid the great shortcoming of similar institutions; and in asking the working man for his confidence, to set him the great example and give him theirs in return. You will judge for yourselves if I promise too much for the working man, when I say that he will stand by such an enterprise with the utmost of his patience, his perseverance, sense, and support; that I am sure he will need no charitable aid or condescending patronage; but will readily and cheerfully pay for the advantages which it confers; that he will prepare himself in individual cases where he feels that the adverse circumstances around him have rendered it necessary; in a word, that he will feel his responsibility like an honest man, and will most honestly and manfully discharge it. I now proceed to the pleasant task to which I assure you I have looked forward for a long time.

26. Based upon the contextual evidence provided in the passage above, what is the meaning of the term *enterprise* in the third paragraph?
    a. Company
    b. Courage
    c. Game
    d. Cause

27. The speaker addresses his audience as *My Good Friends*—what kind of credibility does this salutation give to the speaker?
    a. The speaker is an employer addressing his employees, so the salutation is a way for the boss to bridge the gap between himself and his employees.
    b. The speaker's salutation is one from an entertainer to his audience and uses the friendly language to connect to his audience before a serious speech.
    c. The salutation gives the serious speech that follows a somber tone, as it is used ironically.
    d. The speech is one from a politician to the public, so the salutation is used to grab the audience's attention.

28. According to the aforementioned passage, what is the speaker's second desire for his time in front of the audience?
    a. To read a Christmas story
    b. For the working man to have a say in his institution which is designed for his benefit.
    c. To have an opportunity to stand in their presence
    d. For the life of the institution to be essential to the audience as a whole

Questions 29–32 refer to the following passage:

> Although many Missourians know that Harry S. Truman and Walt Disney hailed from their great state, probably far fewer know that it was also home to the remarkable George Washington Carver. At the end of the Civil War, Moses Carver, the slave owner who owned George's parents, decided to keep George and his brother and raise them on his farm. As a child, George was driven to learn and he loved painting. He even went on to study art while in college but was encouraged to pursue botany instead. He spent much of his life helping others by showing them better ways to farm; his ideas improved agricultural productivity in many countries. One of his most notable contributions to the newly emerging class of Negro farmers was to teach them the negative effects of agricultural monoculture, i.e. growing the same crops in the same fields year after year, depleting the soil of much needed nutrients and resulting in a lesser yielding crop. Carver was an innovator, always thinking of new and better ways to do things, and is most famous for his over three hundred uses for the peanut. Toward the end of his career, Carver returned to his first love of art. Through his artwork, he hoped to inspire people to see the beauty around them and to do great things themselves. When Carver died, he left his money to help fund ongoing agricultural research. Today, people still visit and study at the George Washington Carver Foundation at Tuskegee Institute.

29. Which of the following describes the kind of writing used in the above passage?
    a. Narrative
    b. Persuasive
    c. Technical
    d. Expository

30. According to the passage, what was George Washington Carver's first love?
    a. Plants
    b. Art
    c. Animals
    d. Soil

31. According to the passage, what is the best definition for agricultural monoculture?
    a. The practice of producing or growing a single crop or plant species over a wide area and for a large number of consecutive years
    b. The practice of growing a diversity of crops and rotating them from year to year
    c. The practice of growing crops organically to avoid the use of pesticides
    d. The practice of charging an inflated price for cheap crops to obtain a greater profit margin

32. Which of the following is the best summary of this passage?
    a. George Washington Carver was born at a time when scientific discovery was at a virtual standstill.
    b. Because he was African American, there were not many opportunities for George Washington Carver.
    c. George Washington Carver was an intelligent man whose research and discoveries had an impact worldwide.
    d. George Washington Carver was far more successful as an artist than he was as a scientist.

Questions 33–37 are based upon the following passage:

This excerpt is adaptation from *The Life-Story of Insects,* by Geo H. Carpenter.

> Insects as a whole are preeminently creatures of the land and the air. This is shown not only by the possession of wings by a vast majority of the class, but by the mode of breathing to which reference has already been made, a system of branching air-tubes carrying atmospheric air with its combustion-supporting oxygen to all the insect's tissues. The air gains access to these tubes through a number of paired air-holes or spiracles, arranged segmentally in series.
>
> It is of great interest to find that, nevertheless, a number of insects spend much of their time under water. This is true of not a few in the perfect winged state, as for example aquatic beetles and water-bugs ('boatmen' and 'scorpions') which have some way of protecting their spiracles when submerged, and, possessing usually the power of flight, can pass on occasion from pond or stream to upper air. But it is advisable in connection with our present subject to dwell especially on some insects that remain continually under water till they are ready to undergo their final moult and attain the winged state, which they pass entirely in the air. The preparatory instars of such insects are aquatic; the adult instar is aerial. All may-flies, dragon-flies, and caddis-flies, many beetles and two-winged flies, and a few moths thus divide their life-story between the water and the air. For the present we confine attention to the Stone-flies, the May-flies, and the

Dragon-flies, three well-known orders of insects respectively called by systematists the Plecoptera, the Ephemeroptera and the Odonata.

In the case of many insects that have aquatic larvae, the latter are provided with some arrangement for enabling them to reach atmospheric air through the surface-film of the water. But the larva of a stone-fly, a dragon-fly, or a may-fly is adapted more completely than these for aquatic life; it can, by means of gills of some kind, breathe the air dissolved in water.

33. Which statement best details the central idea in this passage?
   a. It introduces certain insects that transition from water to air.
   b. It delves into entomology, especially where gills are concerned.
   c. It defines what constitutes as insects' breathing.
   d. It invites readers to have a hand in the preservation of insects.

34. Which definition most closely relates to the usage of the word *moult* in the passage?
   a. An adventure of sorts, especially underwater
   b. Mating act between two insects
   c. The act of shedding part or all of the outer shell
   d. Death of an organism that ends in a revival of life

35. What is the purpose of the first paragraph in relation to the second paragraph?
   a. The first paragraph serves as a cause and the second paragraph serves as an effect.
   b. The first paragraph serves as a contrast to the second.
   c. The first paragraph is a description for the argument in the second paragraph.
   d. The first and second paragraphs are merely presented in a sequence.

36. What does the following sentence most nearly mean?
   The preparatory instars of such insects are aquatic; the adult instar is aerial.

   a. The volume of water is necessary to prep the insect for transition rather than the volume of the air.
   b. The abdomen of the insect is designed like a star in the water as well as the air.
   c. The stage of preparation in between molting is acted out in the water, while the last stage is in the air.
   d. These insects breathe first in the water through gills yet continue to use the same organs to breathe in the air.

37. Which of the statements reflect information that one could reasonably infer based on the author's tone?
   a. The author's tone is persuasive and attempts to call the audience to action.
   b. The author's tone is passionate due to excitement over the subject and personal narrative.
   c. The author's tone is informative and exhibits interest in the subject of the study.
   d. The author's tone is somber, depicting some anger at the state of insect larvae.

Random Lake Advertisement

> Who needs the hassle of traveling far away? This summer, why not rent a house on Random Lake? Located conveniently ten miles away from Random City, Random Lake has everything a family needs. Swimming, kayaking, boating, fishing, volleyball, mini-golf, go-cart track, eagle watching, nature trails—there are enough activities here to keep a family busy for a month, much less a week.
>
> Random Lake hotels are available for every lifestyle and budget. Prefer a pool or free breakfast? Prefer quiet? Historical? Modern? No problem. The Random Lake area has got you covered. House rentals are affordable too. During the summer months, rentals can go as cheaply as 600 dollars a week. Even better deals can be found during the off season. Most homes come fully furnished, and pontoon boats, kayaks, and paddle boats are available for rental. With the Legends and the Broadmoor developments slated for grand openings in March, the choices are endless!

38. The main purpose of this passage is to do what?
    a. Describe
    b. Inform
    c. Persuade
    d. Entertain

39. Which of the following sentences is out of place and should be removed?
    a. "This summer, why not rent a house on Random Lake?"
    b. "There are enough activities here to keep a family busy for a month."
    c. "Pontoon boats, kayaks, and paddle boats are available for rental."
    d. "With several new housing developments slated for grand opening in March, the choices are endless!"

40. Which of the following can be deduced from Passages 1 and 2?
    a. Random City is more populated than Random Lake.
    b. The Random Lake area is newer than Random City.
    c. The Random Lake area is growing.
    d. Random Lake prefers families to couples.

Questions 41–45 are based upon the following passage:

This excerpt is adaptation from "What to the Slave is the Fourth of July?" Rochester, New York, July 5, 1852.

> Fellow citizens—Pardon me, and allow me to ask, why am I called upon to speak here today? What have I, or those I represent, to do with your national independence? Are the great principles of political freedom and of natural justice embodied in that Declaration of Independence, Independence extended to us? And am I therefore called upon to bring our humble offering to the national altar, and to confess the benefits, and express devout gratitude for the blessings, resulting from your independence to us?

Would to God, both for your sakes and ours, ours that an affirmative answer could be truthfully returned to these questions! Then would my task be light, and my burden easy and delightful. For who is there so cold that a nation's sympathy could not warm him? Who so obdurate and dead to the claims of gratitude, gratitude that that would not thankfully acknowledge such priceless benefits? Who so stolid and selfish, that would not give his voice to swell the hallelujahs of a nation's jubilee, when the chains of servitude had been torn from his limbs? I am not that man. In a case like that, the dumb may eloquently speak, and the lame man leap as an hart.

But, such is not the state of the case. I say it with a sad sense of the disparity between us. I am not included within the pale of this glorious anniversary. Oh pity! Your high independence only reveals the immeasurable distance between us. The blessings in which you this day rejoice, I do not enjoy in common. The rich inheritance of justice, liberty, prosperity, and independence, bequeathed by your fathers, is shared by *you*, not by *me*. This Fourth of July is *yours,* not *mine*. You may rejoice, *I* must mourn. To drag a man in fetters into the grand illuminated temple of liberty, and call upon him to join you in joyous anthems, were inhuman mockery and sacrilegious irony. Do you mean, citizens, to mock me, by asking me to speak today? If so there is a parallel to your conduct. And let me warn you that it is dangerous to copy the example of a nation whose crimes, towering up to heaven, were thrown down by the breath of the Almighty, burying that nation and irrecoverable ruin! I can today take up the plaintive lament of a peeled and woe-smitten people.

By the rivers of Babylon, there we sat down. Yea! We wept when we remembered Zion. We hanged our harps upon the willows in the midst thereof. For there, they that carried us away captive, required of us a song; and they who wasted us required of us mirth, saying, "Sing us one of the songs of Zion." How can we sing the Lord's song in a strange land? If I forget thee, O Jerusalem, let my right hand forget her cunning. If I do not remember thee, let my tongue cleave to the roof of my mouth.

41. What is the tone of the first paragraph of this passage?
    a. Exasperated
    b. Inclusive
    c. Contemplative
    d. Nonchalant

42. Which word CANNOT be used synonymously with the term *obdurate* as it is conveyed in the text below?

    Who so obdurate and dead to the claims of gratitude, that would not thankfully acknowledge such priceless benefits?

    a. Steadfast
    b. Stubborn
    c. Contented
    d. Unwavering

43. What is the central purpose of this text?
    a. To demonstrate the author's extensive knowledge of the Bible
    b. To address the feelings of exclusion expressed by African Americans after the establishment of the Fourth of July holiday
    c. To convince wealthy landowners to adopt new holiday rituals
    d. To explain why minorities often relished the notion of segregation in government institutions

44. Which statement serves as evidence of the question above?
    a. By the rivers of Babylon . . . down.
    b. Fellow citizens . . . today.
    c. I can . . . woe-smitten people.
    d. The rich inheritance of justice . . . *not by me.*

45. The statement below features an example of which of the following literary devices?
    Oh pity! Your high independence only reveals the immeasurable distance between us.

    a. Assonance
    b. Parallelism
    c. Amplification
    d. Hyperbole

Questions 46–49 are based on the following passage:

The more immediately after the commission of a crime a punishment is inflicted, the more just and useful it will be. It will be more just, because it spares the criminal the cruel and superfluous torment of uncertainty, which increases in proportion to the strength of his imagination and the sense of his weakness; and because the privation of liberty, being a punishment, ought to be inflicted before condemnation, but for as short a time as possible. Imprisonments, I say, being only the means of securing the person of the accused, until he be tried, condemned, or acquitted, ought not only to be of as short duration, but attended with as little severity as possible. The time should be determined by the necessary preparation for the trial, and the right of priority in the oldest prisoners. The confinement ought not to be closer than is requisite to prevent his flight, or his concealing the proofs of the crime; and the trial should be conducted with all possible expedition. Can there be a more cruel contrast than that between the indolence of a judge, and the painful anxiety of the accused; the comforts and pleasures of an insensible magistrate, and the filth and misery of the prisoner? In general, as I have before observed, *the degree of the punishment, and the consequences of a crime, ought to be so contrived, as to have the greatest possible effect on others, with the least possible pain to the delinquent.* If there be any society in which this is not a fundamental principle, it is an unlawful society; for mankind, by their union, originally intended to subject themselves to the least evils possible.

An immediate punishment is more useful; because the smaller the interval of time between the punishment and the crime, the stronger and more lasting will be the association of the two ideas of *Crime* and *Punishment;* so that they may be considered, one as the cause, and the other as the unavoidable and necessary effect. It is demonstrated, that the association of ideas is the cement which unites the fabric of the human intellect; without which, pleasure and pain would be simple and ineffectual sensations. The vulgar, that is, all men who have no general ideas or universal principles, act in consequence of the most immediate and familiar associations; but the more remote and complex only present themselves to the minds of those who are passionately attached to a single object, or to those of greater understanding, who have acquired an habit of rapidly comparing together a number of objects, and of forming a conclusion; and the result, that is, the action in consequence, by these means, becomes less dangerous and uncertain.

It is, then, of the greatest importance, that the punishment should succeed the crime as immediately as possible, if we intend, that, in the rude minds of the multitude, the seducing picture of the advantage arising from the crime, should instantly awake the attendant idea of punishment. Delaying the punishment serves only to separate these two ideas; and thus affects the minds of the spectators rather as being a terrible sight than the necessary consequence of a crime; the horror of which should contribute to heighten the idea of the punishment.

There is another excellent method of strengthening this important connexion between the ideas of crime and punishment; that is, to make the punishment as analogous as possible to the nature of the crime; in order that the punishment may lead the mind to consider the crime in a different point of view, from that in which it was placed by the flattering idea of promised advantages.

Crimes of less importance are commonly punished, either in the obscurity of a prison, or the criminal is *transported*, to give, by his slavery, an example to societies which he never offended; an example absolutely useless, because distant from the place where the crime was committed. Men do not, in general, commit great crimes deliberately, but rather in a sudden gust of passion; and they commonly look on the punishment due to a great crime as remote and improbable. The public punishment, therefore, of small crimes will make a greater impression, and, by deterring men from the smaller, will effectually prevent the greater.

(Cesare Beccaria, "Punishments, Advantages of Immediate," *The Criminal Recorder,* 1810).

46. What is the main purpose of this passage?
    a. To describe
    b. To inform
    c. To persuade
    d. To entertain

47. What text structure is this passage using?
    a. Compare/contrast
    b. Sequential
    c. Cause/effect
    d. Problem-solution

48. Which of the following excerpts best exemplifies the main idea of this passage?
    a. "The vulgar, that is, all men who have no general ideas or universal principles, act in consequence of the most immediate and familiar associations."
    b. "Crimes of less importance are commonly punished, either in the obscurity of a prison, or the criminal is *transported*, to give, by his slavery, an example to societies which he never offended."
    c. "Men do not, in general, commit great crimes deliberately, but rather in a sudden gust of passion; and they commonly look on the punishment due to a great crime as remote and improbable."
    d. "The more immediately after the commission of a crime a punishment is inflicted, the more just and useful it will be."

49. With which of the following statements would the author most likely disagree?
    a. Criminals are incapable of connecting crime and punishment.
    b. A punishment should quickly follow the crime.
    c. Most criminals do not think about the consequences of their actions.
    d. Where a criminal is punished is just as important as when.

Vocabulary

1. What word meaning "harshly criticizing" best fits in the following sentence? The charge nurse was fired for frequently _____ the staff.
    a. Macerating
    b. Extoling
    c. Lauding
    d. Denigrating

2. Select the correct meaning of the underlined word in the following sentence. The patient's cheeks appeared <u>ruddy</u>.
    a. Swollen or puffy
    b. Edematous
    c. Flushed
    d. Discolored or blotchy

3. What word meaning "to infer" best fits in the following sentence? The nurse was able to _____ that the patient was allergic to the ointment.
    a. Deduce
    b. Induce
    c. Conjecture
    d. Construct

4. What word meaning "unexpected and unfortunate" best fits in the following sentence? It was _____ circumstances that landed the patient in the ER.
    a. Adversary
    b. Untoward
    c. Undulated
    d. Unobstructed

5. What is the best definition of the word *chorea*?
    a. A digestive condition common in infants
    b. An abnormal discharge from any body orifice, particularly the ears or eyes
    c. Any disorder of the nervous system that includes involuntary, jerky movements
    d. Weakness of the peripheral muscles

6. Select the correct meaning of the underlined word in the following sentence. The nurse informed the toddler's mother that the boy should start to sleep better once the cause of his <u>pruritis</u> was identified and treated.
    a. Vomiting
    b. Ringing in the ears
    c. Insomnia
    d. Itchiness

7. What word meaning "on the same side" best fits in the following sentence? The patient complained of _____ shoulder and wrist pain.
   a. Bilateral
   b. Ipsilateral
   c. Contralateral
   d. Alateral

8. Select the correct meaning of the underlined word in the following sentence. The medication side effects that the patient experienced were <u>diaphoresis</u> and dizziness.
   a. Excessive sweating
   b. Dyspnea
   c. Wheezing
   d. Frequent urination

9. Select the correct meaning of the underlined word in the following sentence. The nurse explained the risk factors for contracting a <u>venereal</u> disease.
   a. Vector-borne
   b. Sexually-transmitted
   c. Relating to the gums
   d. Parasitic

10. What word meaning "to renounce" best fits in the following sentence? After witnessing the consequences of smoking on his dental health, the patient decided to _____ his beliefs that smoking was harmless.
   a. Abstain
   b. Inculcate
   c. Abjure
   d. Interrogate

11. What is the best definition of the word *deleterious*?
   a. Removable
   b. Excision
   c. Harmful
   d. Deferable

12. What word meaning "inability to feel pleasure" best fits in the following sentence? The nurse referred the patient to a psychologist on account of his insomnia and _____.
   a. Athetosis
   b. Depression
   c. Contentment
   d. Anhedonia

13. Select the correct meaning of the underlined word in the following sentence. The doctor studied the newborn's face for <u>nuances</u> in expression.
   a. Apparent disparities
   b. Subtle differences
   c. Drastic changes
   d. Visual cues

14. What word meaning "further from the trunk" best fits in the following sentence? The ankle is
_____ to the knee.
   a. Dorsal
   b. Distal
   c. Proximal
   d. Ventral

15. What word meaning "apathetic" or "composed" best fits in the following sentence? The _____ demeanor of the patient made it difficult to read his true level of pain.
   a. Egregious
   b. Insolent
   c. Impervious
   d. Phlegmatic

16. What word meaning "caused or produced by an agent outside the body" best fits in the following sentence? Use of _____ testosterone had reduced his body's ability to produce the hormone.
   a. Steroid
   b. Organic
   c. Exogenous
   d. Endogenous

17. Select the correct meaning of the underlined word in the following sentence. The surgeon was concerned about the patient's prognosis.
   a. Outlook
   b. Etiology
   c. Mechanism of transmission
   d. Incidence in the population

18. What word meaning "body wasting usually due to chronic illness" best fits in the following sentence? Over time, it became clear that her uncontrolled AIDS had caused _____.
   a. Catatonia
   b. Anorexia
   c. Ataxia
   d. Cachexia

19. What is the best definition of the word *palpate*?
   a. Fluttering
   b. An abnormal heartbeat
   c. To physically examine using touch
   d. To splint or support a body part

20. Select the correct meaning of the underlined word in the following sentence. The patient with the transtibial amputation used crutches as an auxiliary aid.
   a. Relating to the armpit
   b. Prosthetic
   c. Ambulatory
   d. Ancillary

21. What word meaning "innocent" best fits in the following sentence? The young child's _____ expression was sweet and endearing.
    a. Guileless
    b. Cunning
    c. Begrudging
    d. Vapid

22. What is the best definition of the word *vacuous*?
    a. Inane
    b. A cellular organelle
    c. Suction
    d. Ingenious

23. Select the correct meaning of the underlined word in the following sentence. The charge nurse was a good leader because she had gravitas and commanded respect.
    a. Intelligence
    b. Dignity
    c. Gratitude
    d. Somberness

24. What word meaning "sticking together of membranous surfaces" best fits in the following sentence? The biker had _____ along his scar tissue.
    a. Adhesions
    b. Abrasions
    c. Contusions
    d. Avulsions

25. Select the correct meaning of the underlined word in the following sentence. An ultrasound was ordered to image the patient's hepatic portal system.
    a. Relating to the pancreas
    b. Relating to the liver
    c. Relating to the kidney
    d. Relating to gallbladder

26. What is the best definition of the word *peritoneum*?
    a. The smooth muscular contractions that propel food along the digestive tract
    b. The region between the anus and scrotum
    c. The outer connective tissue layer covering bones
    d. The serous membrane lining the abdominal cavity

27. Select the correct meaning of the underlined word in the following sentence. The vehement speeches from former patients motivated many donors to increase their pledges.
    a. Ardent
    b. Motivational
    c. Novel
    d. Virulent

28. What word meaning "the space inside a hollow or tubular structure" best fits in the following sentence? The atherosclerotic plaques decreased the volume of the arterial _____.
   a. Lumen
   b. Constriction
   c. Angioplasty
   d. Vessel

29. What word meaning "confused" best fits in the following sentence? Upon waking from the procedure, the patient was _____.
   a. Lucid
   b. Anesthetized
   c. Befuddled
   d. Diffident

30. Select the medical term for a "bed sore."
   a. Decubitus ulcer
   b. Duodenal ulcer
   c. Neurotropic ulcer
   d. Ischemic ulcer

31. What word meaning to "conduct towards something" best fits in the following sentence? The _____ nerve carried the signal from the receptor to the spinal cord.
   a. Stimuli
   b. Interneuron
   c. Efferent
   d. Afferent

32. What is the best definition of the word *eschar*?
   a. Scar tissue
   b. Skin ulcer
   c. Dark scab
   d. Fistula

33. What is the best definition of the word *pallor*?
   a. Turgor
   b. Flushed skin
   c. Wan
   d. Febrile

34. What is the best definition of the word *rhinorrhea*?
   a. Nasal discharge
   b. Sinus pressure
   c. Sneezing
   d. Nosebleed

35. Select the correct meaning of the underlined word in the following sentence. The medication had an intrathecal route of administration.
    a. Under tongue
    b. Around the spinal cord
    c. In the ear
    d. Inside the cheek

36. What is the best definition of the word *lament*?
    a. Verbally express grief
    b. Reconcile
    c. Encourage
    d. Verbally extol

37. What is the best definition of the word *noxious*?
    a. Relating to oxygen
    b. Innocuous
    c. Irritating
    d. Harmful

38. What is the best definition of the word *kyphosis*?
    a. An abnormal lateral curvature of the spine
    b. An inward curvature of the cervical spine
    c. An outward curvature of the thoracic spine
    d. Swayback or the commonly seen excessive curvature of the lumbar spine

39. Select the correct meaning of the underlined word in the following sentence. The graduate student's thesis was focused on gerontology.
    a. The study of diseases
    b. The study of growth
    c. The study of genes
    d. The study of aging

40. For which suspected condition might an endoscopy be ordered?
    a. Ulcerative colitis
    b. Peptic ulcer
    c. Angina
    d. Pulmonary embolism

41. What word meaning "uncompromising" best fits in the following sentence? The patient remained _____ in his refusal to take medications.
    a. Intransigent
    b. Complacent
    c. Inexplicable
    d. Confound

42. Blood pressure would be recorded as which of the following?
    a. Subjective data
    b. Objective data
    c. Assessment
    d. Plan

43. What is a terminal illness?
   a. One from which a patient will likely not recover
   b. The most recent illness a patient had
   c. One that is not infectious
   d. One that the patient is born with

44. Where is the popliteal fossa located?
   a. The knee
   b. The skull
   c. The hip
   d. The scapula

45. What word meaning "a model of perfection" best fits in the following sentence? Her chart notes were a _____ of medical records.
   a. Parable
   b. Paradox
   c. Paragon
   d. Paraphrase

46. Select the correct meaning of the underlined word in the following sentence. The hospital room looked pristine.
   a. Unorganized and dingy
   b. Unfriendly
   c. Sterile
   d. Clean and new

47. What is tinnitus?
   a. Ringing in the ear
   b. Temporary deafness
   c. Grinding the teeth
   d. Clicking jaw

48. What does the suffix -itis mean?
   a. Pain
   b. Disease
   c. Inflammation
   d. Tumor

49. What is dysphagia?
   a. Difficulty breathing
   b. Difficulty recognizing faces
   c. Difficulty swallowing
   d. Difficulty speaking

50. What is urticaria?
   a. Burning urine
   b. Kidney stones
   c. Bladder infection
   d. Hives

Grammar

1. Which sentence is grammatically correct?
    a. The baseball that is autographed belongs to whom?
    b. The baseball which is autographed belongs to who?
    c. Whom does the baseball which is autographed belong to?
    d. Whom does the baseball that is autographed belong to?

2. Which of the following words is spelled incorrectly?
    a. Caffiene
    b. Counterfeit
    c. Sleigh
    d. Receipt

3. Which sentence is grammatically incorrect?
    a. Will you please bring me the water before you take her the pizza?
    b. Can I put the box on the shelf where you can reach?
    c. Will you lend me your pen so I can sign for my loan?
    d. What if the two of us were to gather too many flowers?

4. Which word combination properly completes the following sentence?
    I hurt my ankle_____ but now it feels _____.
    a. badly/good
    b. bad/good
    c. bad/well
    d. badly/well

5. Which of the following sentences is a fragment?
    a. We went to the zoo to see the tigers and lions.
    b. Instead we saw elephants, zebras and giraffes.
    c. Because the lion and tiger habitat was closed.
    d. What sound does a giraffe make anyway?

6. Which of the following is a run-on sentence?
    a. I love to go water-skiing, I love alpine skiing, I also love Nordic skiing.
    b. The best way to learn to ski is to take lessons.
    c. All three types of skiing require different skills and different equipment.
    d. It takes a long time to learn how to ski; waterskiing takes the longest time.

7. Which sentence has a dangling modifier?
    a. Eating a large meal, I had to chew my food slowly.
    b. Eating a large meal, my food had to be chewed slowly.
    c. Eating a large meal, I was too full afterward.
    d. Eating a large meal, I was more full than I have ever been.

8. Which of the following choices is an example of a double comparison?
   a. More attainable
   b. Most excited
   c. Most impossible
   d. Less fortunate

9. Which sentence uses a passive voice?
   a. Anna gave the necklace away.
   b. The necklace was given away.
   c. Anna was given the necklace.
   d. The necklace was given away by Anna.

10. Which choice is the future perfect tense of the base word hope?
    a. Hope
    b. Will have hoped
    c. Hoped
    d. Will hope

11. Which sentence is an example of a double negative?
    a. She couldn't find anything to say.
    b. He did like something she said.
    c. They didn't like nothing I said.
    d. I cannot say I don't disapprove of that.

12. What is the subject complement in the following sentence?
    Pulling heavy rope helps strengthen muscles.
    a. Heavy rope
    b. Muscles
    c. Strengthen
    d. Pulling heavy rope

13. In which sentence is there a correlative conjunction?
    a. Whether Amber went to the game or not didn't matter.
    b. Amber and Amanda went to the game together.
    c. They sat in their car while it was raining.
    d. But they eventually got to see the game.

15. Which version of the following sentence has correct capitalization?
    "i told mother about my favorite book: *all the light we cannot see,*" said martha. "she liked it."
    a. "i Told mother about my Favorite Book: *all the light we cannot see,*" Said martha. "she Liked it.
    b. "I told mother about my favorite Book: *All The Light We Cannot See,*" Said Martha. "she liked it."
    c. "I told Mother about my favorite book: *All the Light We Cannot See,*" said Martha. "She liked it."
    d. I told Mother about my favorite book: ALL THE LIGHT WE CANNOT SEE," said Martha. "She liked it."

16. Which sentence below is punctuated correctly with periods?
    a. It's 2 pm and I've forgotten my appointment with Dr Samson
    b. It's 2PM and I've forgotten my appointment with Dr. Samson
    c. It's 2 P.M. and I've forgotten my appointment with Dr. Samson.
    d. It's 2 P.M. and I've forgotten. my appointment with Dr Samson.

17. Which sentence below is punctuated correctly with a question mark?
    a. Can you please take the garbage out?
    b. I wonder if anyone has taken the garbage out?
    c. Miles asked Lisa if she'd taken out the garbage?
    d. Didn't anybody take the garbage out?

18. Which sentence below is punctuated correctly with an exclamation mark?
    a. Can you eat more than one slice of pizza!
    b. Yikes! That startled me!
    c. The cow jumped over the moon?!
    d. That's impossible!!!!!

19. Which sentence below is punctuated correctly with commas?
    a. The sample consisted of several cheeses, two, meats, and three, crackers.
    b. Mother Teresa, a humanitarian, said, "Be kind to one another."
    c. Hello friend, how have you been, lately?
    d. He ate too much food, consequently, he had a stomachache and heartburn.

20. Which sentence is punctuated correctly with colons and semicolons?
    a. There are four people who are most important to me; my husband Harold; my daughter Sarah; my friend Debbie; and my sister Jenna.
    b. There are four people; who are most important to me: my husband Harold, my daughter Sarah, my friend Debbie, and my sister Jenna.
    c. There are four people who are most important to me; my husband: Harold, my daughter: Sarah, my friend: Debbie, and my sister: Jenna
    d. There are four people who are most important to me: my husband, Harold; my daughter, Sarah; my friend, Debbie; and my sister, Jenna.

21. Which quotation is punctuated correctly?
    a. Daniel said, "I want to travel to Mars."
    b. Daniel said "I want to travel to Mars".
    c. Daniel said, I want to "travel to Mars".
    d. "Daniel said I want to travel to Mars."

22. Which subject/verb agreement makes the following sentence grammatically correct?
    The _____ _____ at the championship on March 7ᵗʰ.
    a. teams/competes
    b. teams/wins
    c. team/competes
    d. team/win

23. Which sentence shows grammatically correct subject/verb agreement?
    a. The professor of physics compliments the student.
    b. The professor of physics compliment the student.
    c. The professors of physics compliments the student.
    d. The professors of physics will compliments the student.

24. Which sentence below does not contain an error in comma usage for dates?
    a. My niece arrives from Australia on Monday, February 4, 2016.
    b. My cousin's wedding this Saturday June 9, conflicts with my best friend's birthday party.
    c. The project is due on Tuesday, May, 17, 2016.
    d. I can't get a flight home until Thursday September 21.

25. Which of the following sentences uses correct spelling?
    a. Although he believed himself to be a consciensious judge of character, his judgment in this particular situation was grossly erroneous.
    b. Although he believed himself to be a conscientious judge of character, his judgment in this particular situation was grossly erroneous.
    c. Although he believed himself to be a conscientious judge of character, his judgement in this particular situation was grossly erroneous.
    d. Although he believed himself to be a concientious judge of character, his judgemant in this particular situation was grossly erroneous.

26. The stress of preparing for the exam was starting to take its toll on me.

In the preceding sentence, what part of speech is the word *stress*?
    a. Verb
    b. Noun
    c. Adjective
    d. Adverb

27. Select the example that uses the correct plural form.
    a. Rooves
    b. Octopi
    c. Potatos
    d. Fishes

28. Which of these examples uses correct punctuation?
    a. The presenter said, "The award goes to," and my heart skipped a beat.
    b. The presenter said, "The award goes to" and my heart skipped a beat.
    c. The presenter said "The award goes to" and my heart skipped a beat.
    d. The presenter said, "The award goes to", and my heart skipped a beat.

29. Select the sentence in which the word *counter* functions as an adjective.
    a. The kitchen counter was marred and scratched from years of use.
    b. He countered my offer for the car, but it was still much higher than I was prepared to pay.
    c. Her counter argument was very well presented and logically thought out.
    d. Some of the board's proposals ran counter to the administration's policies.

30. In which of the following sentences does the pronoun correctly agree with its antecedent?
    a. Human beings on the planet have the right to his share of clean water, food, and shelter.
    b. Human beings on the planet have the right to their share of clean water, food, and shelter.
    c. Human beings on the planet have the right to its share of clean water, food, and shelter.
    d. Human beings on the planet have the right to her share of clean water, food, and shelter.

31 Every single one of my mother's siblings, their spouses, and their children met in Colorado for a week-long family vacation last summer.

Which of the following is the complete subject of the preceding sentence?
    a. Every single one
    b. Siblings, spouses, children
    c. One
    d. Every single one of my mother's siblings, their spouses, and their children

32. Walking through the heavily wooded park by the river in October, I was amazed at the beautiful colors of the foliage, the bright blue sky, and the crystal-clear water.

Using the context clues in the preceding sentence, which of the following words is the correct meaning of the word foliage?
    a. Leaves of the trees
    b. Feathers of the birds
    c. Tree bark
    d. Rocks on the path

33. Which of the following sentences incorrectly uses italics?
    a. *Old Yeller* is a classic in children's literature, yet very few young people today have read it or even seen the movie.
    b. My favorite musical of all time has to be *The Sound of Music* followed closely by *Les Miserables.*
    c. Langston Hughes's famous poem *Dreams* is the most anthologized of all his works.
    d. When I went to the Louvre, I was surprised at how small Leonardo de Vinci's *Mona Lisa* is compared to other paintings.

34. Which of the following sentences employs correct usage?
    a. It's always a better idea to ask permission first rather than ask for forgiveness later.
    b. Its always a better idea to ask permission first rather than ask for forgiveness later.
    c. It's always a better idea to ask permission first rather then ask for forgiveness later.
    d. Its always a better idea to ask permission first rather then ask for forgiveness later.

35. Which of the following is an imperative sentence?
    a. The state flower of Texas is the blue bonnet.
    b. Do you know if the team is playing in the finals or not?
    c. Take the first right turn, and then go one block west.
    d. We won in overtime!

36. Identify the compound sentence from the following examples:
    a. John and Adam met for coffee before going to class.
    b. As I was leaving, my dad called and needed to talk.
    c. I ran before work and went to the gym afterward for an hour or so.
    d. Felix plays the guitar in my roommate's band, and Alicia is the lead vocalist.

37. Jose had three exams on Monday, so he spent several hours in the library the day before and more time in his dorm room that night studying.

Identify all the words that function as nouns in the preceding sentence:
   a. Jose, exams, hours, library, day, time, room, night
   b. Jose, exams, Monday, hours, library, day, time, room, night
   c. Jose, exams, Monday, he, hours, library, day, time, dorm, night
   d. Exams, Monday, hours, library, day, time, room, night

38. Identify the sentence that uses correct subject-verb agreement.
   a. Each of the students have completed the final project and presentation.
   b. Many players on the basketball team was injured in last night's game.
   c. My friends from school has been trying to talk me in to dance classes.
   d. Everyone in my family has broken a bone except for me.

39. Which of the following sentences has an error in capitalization?
   a. My Mom used to live on the East Coast.
   b. I registered for one semester of Famous Women in Film, but there is not enough room in my schedule.
   c. I prefer traveling on Southwest Airlines because they do not charge baggage fees.
   d. I have never been to Martha's Vineyard or to any other part of New England for that matter.

40. *The exhilarating morning air, combined with the beautiful mountain scenery, inspired me to want to jump right out of bed every morning for a lengthy run.*

From the following words, select one that is used as an adjective in the preceding sentence.
   a. Air
   b. Inspired
   c. Exhilarating
   d. Morning

41. My favorite teacher gave _____ and _____ extra credit on our project.
   a. me, him
   b. he, I
   c. him, I
   d. him, me

42. Which of these sentences uses correct punctuation?
   a. We traveled through six states on our road trip; Texas, New Mexico, Colorado, Wyoming, Utah, and Montana.
   b. We traveled through six states on our road trip: Texas, New Mexico, Colorado, Wyoming, Utah, and Montana.
   c. We traveled through six states on our road trip -- Texas, New Mexico, Colorado, Wyoming, Utah, and Montana.
   d. We traveled through six states on our road trip, Texas, New Mexico, Colorado, Wyoming, Utah, and Montana.

43. Which of the following sentences employs correct usage?
    a. You're going to need to go there to get your backpack from their house.
    b. Your going to need to go there to get you're backpack from their house.
    c. You're going to need to go their to get your backpack from there house.
    d. Your going to need to go their to get you're backpack from there house.

44. Which of the following sentences uses passive voice?
    a. My car was terribly dented by hail during the storm the other night.
    b. My car looked great after the car wash and detailing.
    c. The hail damaged not only my car but the roof of my house as well.
    d. The storm rolled through during the night, taking everyone by surprise.

45. Which of the following sentences correctly uses an apostrophe?
    a. The childrens' choir performed at the Music Hall on Tuesday.
    b. The Smith's went to Colorado with us last summer.
    c. The Joneses' house is currently unoccupied while they are out of the country.
    d. Peoples' attitudes about politics are sometimes apathetic.

46. Which of the following sentences uses incorrect parallel structure?
    a. We worked out every day by swimming, biking, and a run.
    b. The list of craft supplies included scissors, glue, tissue paper, and glitter.
    c. Before I can come over, I need to run to the bank, go to the grocery store, and stop by the dry cleaners.
    d. I love to eat good food, take long walks, and read great books.

Directions for questions 47–50: Rewrite the sentence in your head following the directions given below. Keep in mind that your new sentence should be well written and should have essentially the same meaning as the original sentence.

47. Although she was nervous speaking in front of a crowd, the author read her narrative with poise and confidence.

Rewrite, beginning with

<u>The author had poise and confidence while reading</u>

The next words will be
    a. because she was nervous speaking in front of a crowd.
    b. but she was nervous speaking in front of a crowd.
    c. even though she was nervous speaking in front of a crowd.
    d. before she was nervous speaking in front of a crowd.

48. There was a storm surge and loss of electricity during the hurricane.

Rewrite, beginning with: <u>While the hurricane occurred,</u>

The next words will be
    a. there was a storm surge after the electricity went out.
    b. the storm surge caused the electricity to go out.
    c. the electricity surged into the storm.
    d. the electricity went out and there was a storm surge.

49. When one elephant in a herd is sick, the rest of the herd will help it walk and bring it food.

Rewrite, beginning with: <u>An elephant herd will</u>

The next words will be
    a. be too sick and tired to walk
    b. help and support
    c. gather food when they're sick
    d. be unable to walk without food

50. They went out to eat after the soccer game.

Rewrite, beginning with: <u>They finished the soccer game</u>

The next words will be
    a. then went out to eat.
    b. after they went out to eat.
    c. so they could go out to eat.
    d. because they went out to eat.

Biology

1. What types of molecules can move through a cell membrane by passive transport?
    a. Complex sugars
    b. Non-lipid soluble molecules
    c. Oxygen
    d. Molecules moving from areas of low concentration to areas of high concentration

2. What is ONE feature that both prokaryotes and eukaryotes have in common?
    a. A plasma membrane
    b. A nucleus enclosed by a membrane
    c. Organelles
    d. A nucleoid

3. What is the LAST phase of mitosis?
    a. Prophase
    b. Telophase
    c. Anaphase
    d. Metaphase

4. How many daughter cells are formed from one parent cell during meiosis?
    a. One
    b. Two
    c. Three
    d. Four

5. Which base pairs with adenine in RNA?
   a. Thymine
   b. Guanine
   c. Cytosine
   d. Uracil

6. With which genotype would the recessive phenotype appear, if the dominant allele is marked with "A" and the recessive allele is marked with "a"?
   a. AA
   b. aa
   c. Aa
   d. aA

7. What is ONE reason why speciation can occur?
   a. Geographic separation
   b. Seasons
   c. Daylight
   d. A virus

8. What is the broadest, or LEAST specialized, classification of the Linnean taxonomic system?
   a. Species
   b. Family
   c. Domain
   d. Phylum

9. How are fungi similar to plants?
   a. They have a cell wall.
   b. They contain chloroplasts.
   c. They perform photosynthesis.
   d. They use carbon dioxide as a source of energy.

10. What important function are the roots of plants responsible for?
    a. Absorbing water from the surrounding environment
    b. Performing photosynthesis
    c. Conducting sugars downward through the leaves
    d. Supporting the plant body

11. Which of the following would occur in response to a change in water concentration?
    a. Phototropism
    b. Thermotropism
    c. Gravitropism
    d. Hydrotropism

12. Which factor is NOT a consideration in population dynamics?
    a. Size and age of population
    b. Immigration
    c. Hair color
    d. Number of births

13. Which type of diagram describes the cycling of energy and nutrients of an ecosystem?
    a. Food web
    b. Phylogenetic tree
    c. Fossil record
    d. Pedigree chart

14. Which of the following systems does NOT include a transportation system throughout the body?
    a. Cardiovascular system
    b. Endocrine system
    c. Immune system
    d. Nervous system

15. Which of the following correctly identifies a difference between the primary and secondary immune response?
    a. In the secondary response, macrophages migrate to the lymph nodes to present the foreign microorganism to helped T lymphocytes.
    b. The humeral immunity that characterizes the primary response is coordinated by T lymphocytes.
    c. The primary response is quicker and more powerful than the secondary response.
    d. Suppressor T cells activate in the secondary response to prevent an overactive immune response.

16. Which of the following correctly matches a category of protein with a physiologic example?
    a. Keratin is a structural protein
    b. Antigens are hormonal proteins
    c. Channel proteins are marker proteins
    d. Actin is a transport protein

17. Describe the synthesis of the lagging strand of DNA.
    a. DNA polymerases synthesize DNA continuously after initially attaching to a primase.
    b. DNA polymerases synthesize DNA discontinuously in pieces called Okazaki fragments after initially attaching to primases.
    c. DNA polymerases synthesize DNA discontinuously in pieces called Okazaki fragments after initially attaching to RNA primers.
    d. DNA polymerases synthesize DNA discontinuously in pieces called Okazaki fragments which are joined together in the end by a DNA helicase.

18. What is the major difference between somatic and germline mutations?
    a. Somatic mutations usually benefit the individual while germline mutations usually harm them.
    b. Since germline mutations only affect one cell, they are less noticeable than the rapidly dividing somatic cells.
    c. Somatic mutations are not expressed for several generations, but germline mutations are expressed immediately.
    d. Germline mutations are usually inherited while somatic mutations will affect only the individual.

19. Most catalysts found in biological systems are which of the following?
    a. Special lipids called cofactors.
    b. Special proteins called enzymes.
    c. Special lipids called enzymes.
    d. Special proteins called cofactors.

20. Which of the following is directly transcribed from DNA and represents the first step in protein building?

    a. siRNA

    b. rRNA

    c. mRNA

    d. tRNA

21. What information does a genotype give that a phenotype does not?

    a. The genotype necessarily includes the proteins coded for by its alleles.

    b. The genotype will always show an organism's recessive alleles.

    c. The genotype must include the organism's physical characteristics.

    d. The genotype shows what an organism's parents looked like.

	T	t
T		
t		

22. Which statement is supported by the Punnett square above, if "T" = Tall and "t" = short?

    a. Both parents are homozygous tall.

    b. 100% of the offspring will be tall because both parents are tall.

    c. There is a 25% chance that an offspring will be short.

    d. The short allele will soon die out.

23. Which of the following CANNOT be found in a human cell's genes?

    a. Sequences of amino acids to be transcribed into mRNA

    b. Lethal recessive traits like sickle cell anemia

    c. Mutated DNA

    d. DNA that codes for proteins the cell doesn't use

24. A student believes that there is an inverse relationship between sugar consumption and test scores. To test this hypothesis, he recruits several people to eat sugar, wait one hour, and take a short aptitude test afterwards. The student will compile the participants' sugar intake levels and test scores. How should the student conduct the experiment?

    a. One round of testing, where each participant consumes a different level of sugar.

    b. Two rounds of testing: The first, where each participant consumes a different level of sugar, and the second, where each participant consumes the same level as they did in Round 1.

    c. Two rounds of testing: The first, where each participant consumes the same level of sugar as each other, and the second, where each participant consumes the same level of sugar as each other but at higher levels than in Round 1.

    d. One round of testing, where each participant consumes the same level of sugar.

25. Four different groups of the same species of peas are grown and exposed to differing levels of sunlight, water, and fertilizer as documented in the table below. The data in the water and fertilizer columns indicates how many times the peas are watered or fertilized per week, respectively. Group 2 is the only group that withered. What is a reasonable explanation for this occurrence?

Group	Sunlight	Water	Fertilizer
1	partial sun	4 mL/hr	1
2	full sun	7 mL/hr	1
3	no sun	14 mL/hr	2
4	partial sun	3 mL/hr	2

    a. Insects gnawed away the stem of the plant.
    b. The roots rotted due to poor drainage.
    c. The soil type had nutrition deficiencies.
    d. This species of peas does not thrive in full sunlight.

Chemistry

1. Which of following about nuclear reactions is NOT true?
    a. They involve the release of energy
    b. The structure of the nucleus changes.
    c. They take place in the atom's nucleus.
    d. The reactants and products have equal mass.

2. What does the Lewis Dot structure of an element represent?
    a. The outer electron valence shell population
    b. The inner electron valence shell population
    c. The positioning of the element's protons
    d. The positioning of the element's neutrons

3. What is the chemical reaction when a compound is broken down into its elemental components called?
    a. A synthesis reaction
    b. A decomposition reaction
    c. An organic reaction
    d. An oxidation reaction

4. Which of the following is a balanced chemical equation?
    a. $Na + Cl_2 \rightarrow NaCl$
    b. $2Na + Cl_2 \rightarrow NaCl$
    c. $2Na + Cl_2 \rightarrow 2NaCl$
    d. $2Na + 2Cl_2 \rightarrow 2NaCl$

5. What is the name of this compound: CO?
    a. Carbonite oxide
    b. Carbonic dioxide
    c. Carbonic oxide
    d. Carbon monoxide

6. What is the molarity of a solution made by dissolving 4.0 grams of NaCl into enough water to make 120 mL of solution?
    a. 0.34 M
    b. 0.57 M
    c. 0.034 M
    d. 0.057 M

7. Considering a gas in a closed system, at a constant volume, what will happen to the temperature if the pressure is increased?
    a. The temperature will stay the same
    b. The temperature will decrease
    c. The temperature will increase
    d. It cannot be determined with the information given

8. A rock has a mass of 14.3 grams (g) and a volume of 5.4 cm^3, what is its density?
    a. 8.90 g/cm^3
    b. 0.38 g/cm^3
    c. 77.22 g/cm^3
    d. 2.65 g/cm^3

9. Find the lowest coefficients that will balance the following combustion equation.

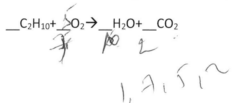

$$\_\_C_2H_{10}+\_\_O_2 \rightarrow \_\_H_2O+\_\_CO_2$$

    a. 1:5:5:2
    b. 4:10:20:8
    c. 2:9:10:4
    d. 2:5:10:4

10. What is the purpose of a catalyst?
    a. To increase a reaction rate by increasing the activation energy
    b. To increase a reaction's rate by increasing the temperature
    c. To increase a reaction's rate by decreasing the activation energy
    d. To increase a reaction's rate by decreasing the temperature

11. Which is NOT a form of Energy?
    a. Light
    b. Sound
    c. Heat
    d. Mass

12. Salts like sodium iodide (NaI) and potassium chloride (KCl) use what type of bond?
    a. Ionic bonds
    b. Disulfide bridges
    c. Covalent bonds
    d. London dispersion forces

13. Which of the following is unique to covalent bonds?
    a. Most covalent bonds are formed between the elements H, F, N, and O.
    b. Covalent bonds are dependent on forming dipoles.
    c. Bonding electrons are shared between two or more atoms.
    d. Molecules with covalent bonds tend to have a crystalline solid structure.

14. Which of the following describes a typical gas?
    a. Indefinite shape and indefinite volume
    b. Indefinite shape and definite volume
    c. Definite shape and definite volume
    d. Definite shape and indefinite volume

15. Which of the following is a chief difference between evaporation and boiling?
    a. Liquids boil only at the surface while they evaporate equally throughout the liquid.
    b. Evaporating substances change from gas to liquid while boiling substances change from liquid to gas.
    c. Evaporation happens in nature while boiling is a manmade phenomenon.
    d. Evaporation can happen below a liquid's boiling point.

16. Which of the following is a special property of water?
    a. Water easily flows through phospholipid bilayers.
    b. A water molecule's oxygen atom allows fish to breathe.
    c. Water is highly cohesive which explains its high melting point.
    d. Water can self-hydrolyze and decompose into hydrogen and oxygen.

17. For any given element, an isotope is an atom with which of the following?
    a. A different atomic number.
    b. A different number of protons.
    c. A different number of electrons.
    d. A different mass number.

18. What is the electrical charge of the nucleus?
    a. A nucleus always has a positive charge.
    b. A stable nucleus has a positive charge, but a radioactive nucleus may have no charge and instead be neutral.
    c. A nucleus always has no charge and is instead neutral.
    d. A stable nucleus has no charge and is instead neutral, but a radioactive nucleus may have a charge.

19. According to the periodic table, which of the following elements is the least reactive?
    a. Fluorine
    b. Silicon
    c. Neon
    d. Gallium

20. Explain the Law of Conservation of Mass as it applies to this reaction: 2H2 + O2 → 2H2O.
    a. Electrons are lost.
    b. The hydrogen loses mass.
    c. New oxygen atoms are formed.
    d. There is no decrease or increase of matter

21. What type of chemical reaction produces a salt?
    a. An oxidation reaction
    b. A neutralization reaction
    c. A synthesis reaction
    d. A decomposition reaction

22. Which of the following correctly displays 8,600,000,000,000 in scientific notation (to two significant figures)?
    a. 8.6×10^{12}
    b. 8.6×10^{-12}
    c. 8.6×10^{11}
    d. 8.60×10^{12}

23. Which of the following best defines the term *amphoteric*?
    a. A substance that conducts electricity due to ionization when dissolved in a solvent
    b. A substance that can act as an acid or a base depending on the properties of the solute
    c. A substance that, according to the Brønsted-Lowry Acid-Base Theory, is a proton-donor
    d. A substance that donates its proton and forms its conjugate base in a neutralization reaction

24. How many grams of solid $CaCO_3$ are needed to make 600 mL of a 0.35 M solution? The atomic masses for the elements are as follows: Ca = 40.07 g/mol; C = 12.01 g/mol; O = 15.99 g/mol.
    a. 18.3 g
    b. 19.7 g
    c. 21.0 g
    d. 24.2 g

25. How many mL (to the appropriate number of significant figures) of a 15.0 M stock solution of HCl should be added to water to create 300 mL of a 1.80 M solution of HCl?
    a. 32.0 mL
    b. 32 mL
    c. 36.0 mL
    d. 36 mL

Anatomy and Physiology

1. What is the order of filtration in the nephron?
    a. Collecting Duct → Proximal tubule → Loop of Henle
    b. Proximal tubule → Loop of Henle → Collecting duct
    c. Loop of Henle → Collecting duct → Proximal tubule
    d. Loop of Henle → Proximal tubule → Collecting duct

2. Which are neurons that transmit signals from the CNS to effector tissues and organs?
    a. Motor
    b. Sensory
    c. Interneuron
    d. Reflex

3. Which statement is NOT true regarding brain structure?
    a. The corpus collosum connects the hemispheres.
    b. Broca and Wernicke's areas are associated with speech and language.
    c. The cerebellum is important for long-term memory storage.
    d. The brainstem is responsible for involuntary movement.

4. Which is NOT a function of the pancreas?
    a. Secretes the hormone insulin in response to growth hormone stimulation
    b. Secretes bicarbonate into the small intestine to raise the pH from stomach secretions
    c. Secretes enzymes used by the small intestine to digest fats, sugars, and proteins
    d. Secretes hormones from its endocrine portion in order to regulate blood sugar levels

5. Which organ is not a component of the lymphatic system?
    a. Thymus
    b. Spleen
    c. Tonsil
    d. Gall bladder

6. Which action is unrelated to blood pH?
    a. Exhalation of carbon dioxide
    b. Kidney reabsorption of bicarbonate
    c. ADH secretion
    d. Nephron secretion of ammonia

7. Which gland regulates calcium levels?
    a. Thyroid
    b. Pineal
    c. Adrenal
    d. Parathyroid

8. What are the functions of the hypothalamus?
        I. Regulate body temperature
        II. Send stimulatory and inhibitory instructions to the pituitary gland
        III. Receives sensory information from the brain
    a. I and II
    b. I and III
    c. II and III
    d. I, II, and III

9. Which muscle system is unlike the others?
    a. Bicep: Tricep
    b. Quadricep: Hamstring
    c. Gluteus maximus: Gluteus minimus
    d. Trapezius/Rhomboids: Pectoralis Major

10. How do muscle fibers shorten during contraction?
    a. The actin filaments attach to the myosin forming cross-bridges and pull the fibers closer together
    b. Calcium enters the sarcoplasmic reticulum, initiating an action potential
    c. Myosin cross-bridges attach, rotate, and detach from actin filaments causing the ends of the sarcomere to be pulled closer together
    d. The t-tubule system allows the fibers to physically shorten during contraction

11. Which of the following is not considered to be a primary function of the proprioceptive system?
    a. Provide awareness of position and kinesthesia within the surroundings
    b. Produce coordinated reflexes to maintain muscle tone and balance
    c. Provide peripheral feedback information to the central nervous system to help modify movements and motor response
    d. Provide cushioning to joints during impact

12. Which of the following correctly explain the order of how muscle spindles sense the rate and magnitude of increasing muscle tension as the muscle lengthens?
    a. The muscle spindle is stretched, sensory neurons in the spindle are activated, an impulse is sent to the spinal cord, motor neurons that innervate extrafusal fibers are signaled to relax
    b. The muscle spindle is stretched, motor neurons in the spindle are activated, an impulse is sent to the spinal cord, sensory neurons that innervate extrafusal fibers are signaled to relax
    c. Sensory neurons in the spindle are activated, the muscle spindle is stretched, an impulse is sent to the spinal cord, motor neurons that innervate extrafusal fibers are signaled to relax
    d. The muscle spindle is stretched, sensory neurons in the spindle are activated, an impulse is sent to the spinal cord, sensory neurons that innervate intrafusal fibers are signaled to relax

13. After assessing a patient's passive range of motion in the knee, the therapist determines there is limitation in flexion. Which of the following list of structures may be responsible for the restricted range of motion?
    a. Quadriceps, ligaments, knee joint capsule, fascia
    b. Hamstrings, ligaments, knee joint capsule, fascia
    c. Gastrocnemius, ligaments, knee joint capsule, fascia
    d. Ligaments, knee joint capsule, fascia

14. Which of the following lists of joint types is in the correct order for increasing amounts of permitted motion (least mobile to most mobile)?
    a. Hinge, condyloid, saddle
    b. Saddle, hinge, condyloid
    c. Saddle, condyloid, hinge
    d. Hinge, saddle, condyloid

15. Which of the following is NOT a component of a sarcomere?
    a. Actin
    b. D-line
    c. B-Band
    d. I-Band

16. Which of the following correctly lists the structures of a muscle from largest to smallest?
    a. Fasciculus, muscle fiber, actin, myofibril
    b. Muscle fiber, fasciculus, myofibril, actin
    c. Sarcomere, fasciculus, myofibril, myosin
    d. Muscle fiber, myofibril, sarcomere, actin

17. Myosin cross-bridges attach reticulum is stimulated to release which of the following?
    a. Calcium ions
    b. Acetylcholine
    c. Troponin
    d. Adenosine triphosphate (ATP)

18. Which of the following types of joints are correctly matched with the anatomic joint example given?
    I. Cartilaginous: pubic symphysis
    II. Saddle: thumb carpal metacarpal
    III. Plane: sutures in skull
    IV. Pivot: radial head on ulna

    a. Choices I, II, III
    b. Choices I, II, IV
    c. Choices I, III, IV
    d. All are correct

19. Which of the following upper body movements take place in the sagittal plane?
    I. Elbow extension
    II. Wrist flexion
    III. Shoulder abduction
    IV. Neck left tilt

    a. I and IV
    b. I, III, IV
    c. I and II
    d. II and III

20. What muscle is the primary antagonist in knee flexion?
    a. Hamstrings
    b. Quadriceps
    c. Gastrocnemius
    d. Tibialis anterior

21. What is the MAIN function of the respiratory system?
    a. To eliminate waste through the kidneys and bladder
    b. To exchange gas between the air and circulating blood
    c. To transform food and liquids into energy
    d. To excrete waste from the body

22. Which system comprises the 206 bones of the body?
    a. Skeletal
    b. Muscular
    c. Endocrine
    d. Reproductive

23. A child complains of heavy breathing even when relaxing. They are an otherwise healthy child with no history of respiratory problems. What might be the issue?
    a. Asthma
    b. Blood clot
    c. Hyperventilation
    d. Exercising too hard

24. Which of the following areas of the body has the most sweat glands?
    a. Upper back
    b. Arms
    c. Feet
    d. Palms

25. Which of the following is the best definition for *genicular?*
    a. Relating to aging
    b. Relating to the knee
    c. Relating to sperm
    d. Relating to the genitals

Physics

1. Which is not a method for transferring electrostatic charge?
    a. Polarization
    b. Touch
    c. Election
    d. Induction

2. What is 45 °C converted to °F?
    a. 113 °F
    b. 135 °F
    c. 57 °F
    d. 88 °F

3. What is the force that opposes motion?
    a. Reactive force
    b. Responsive force
    c. Friction
    d. Momentum

4. Car A (mass 100 kg) traveling at 5 m/s hits Car B (mass 110 kg) traveling at 8 m/s in a head-on collision. The bumpers hook together during the collision so that Car A and Car B travel together after the impact. What is their combined velocity after impact?
    a. 13.0 m/s
    b. 3.0 m/s
    c. 6.6 m/s
    d. 16.6 m/s

5. What is the name of the scale used in sound level meters to measure the intensity of sound waves?
    a. Doppler
    b. Electron
    c. Watt
    d. Decibel

6. According to Newton's Three Laws of Motion, which of the following is true?
    a. Two objects cannot exert a force on each other without touching.
    b. An object at rest has no inertia.
    c. The weight of an object is the same as the mass of the object.
    d. The weight of an object is equal to the mass of an object multiplied by gravity.

7. What effect changes the oscillations of a wave and can alter the appearance of light waves?
    a. Reflection
    b. Refraction
    c. Dispersion
    d. Polarization

8. A spinning ice skater who extends his or her arms horizontally to slow down is demonstrating which of the following?
    a. Conservation of angular momentum
    b. Conservation of mechanical energy
    c. Conservation of matter
    d. Conservation of mass

9. The Sun transferring heat to the Earth through space is an example of which of the following?
    a. Convection
    b. Conduction
    c. Induction
    d. Radiation

10. What is the acceleration of a vehicle starting from rest and reaching a velocity of 15 m/s in 5.0 s?
    a. 3.0 m/s
    b. 75 m/s
    c. 3.0 m/s^2
    d. 75 m/s^2

Answer Explanations

Mathematics

1. B: 300 miles in 4 hours is 300/4 = 75 miles per hour. In 1.5 hours, the car will go 1.5 × 75 miles, or 112.5 miles.

2. C: One apple/orange pair costs $3 total. Therefore, Jan bought 90/3 = 30 total pairs, and hence, she bought 30 oranges.

3. C: The formula for the volume of a box with rectangular sides is the length times width times height, so 5 × 6 × 3 = 90 cubic feet.

4. D: First, the train's journey in the real word is 3 x 50 = 150 miles. On the map, 1 inch corresponds to 10 miles, so there is 150/10 = 15 inches on the map.

5. B: The total trip time is 1 + 3.5 + 0.5 = 5 hours. The total time driving is 1 + 0.5 = 1.5 hours. So, the fraction of time spent driving is 1.5/5 or 3/10. To get the percentage, convert this to a fraction out of 100. The numerator and denominator are multiplied by 10, with a result of 30/100. The percentage is the numerator in a fraction out of 100, so 30%.

6. B: The formula for the volume of a cylinder is $\pi r^2 h$, where r is the radius and h is the height. The diameter is twice the radius, so these barrels have a radius of 1 foot. That means each barrel has a volume of $\pi \times 1^2 \times 3 = 3\pi$ cubic feet. Since there are three of them, the total is $3 \times 3\pi = 9\pi$ cubic feet.

7. A: The tip is not taxed, so he pays 5% tax only on the $10. 5% of $10 is $0.05 \times 10 = \$0.50$. Add up $10 + $2 + $0.50 to get $12.50.

8. A: The first step is to divide up $150 into four equal parts. 150/4 is 37.5, so she needs to save an average of $37.50 per day.

9. D: 300/80 =30/8 = 15/4 =3.75. But Bernard is only working full days, so he will need to work 4 days, since 3 days is not sufficient.

10. A: The value went up by $165,000 – $150,000 = $15,000. Out of $150,000, this is $\frac{15,000}{150,000} = \frac{1}{10}$. Convert this to having a denominator of 100, the result is $\frac{10}{100}$ or 10%.

11. D: The total faculty is 15 + 20 = 35. Therefore, the faculty to student ratio is 35:200. Then, to simplify this ratio, both the numerator and the denominator are divided by 5, since 5 is a common factor of both, which yields 7:40.

12. B: The journey will be 5 × 3 = 15 miles. A car travelling at 60 miles per hour is travelling at 1 mile per minute. So, it will take 15/1 = 15 minutes to take the journey.

13. A: Taylor's total income is $20,000 + $10,000 = $30,000. 15% of this is $\frac{15}{100} = \frac{3}{20}$. So $\frac{3}{20} \times \$30,000 = \frac{90,000}{20} = \frac{9000}{2} = \$4500$.

14. B: Since the answer will be in cubic feet rather than inches, the first step is to convert from inches to feet for the dimensions of the box. There are 12 inches per foot, so the box is 24/12 = 2 feet wide, 18/12 = 1.5 feet deep, and 12/12 = 1 foot high. The volume is the product of these three together: $2 \times 1.5 \times 1 = 3$ cubic feet.

15. D: Kristen bought four DVDs, which would cost a total of $4 \times 15 = \$60$. She spent a total of $100, so she spent $100 – $60 = $40 on CDs. Since they cost $10 each, she must have purchased 40/10 = four CDs.

16. D: This problem can be solved by setting up a proportion involving the given information and the unknown value. The proportion is $\frac{21\ pages}{4\ nights} = \frac{140\ pages}{x\ nights}$. Solving the proportion by cross-multiplying, the equation becomes $21x = 4 * 140$, where $x = 26.67$. Since it is not an exact number of nights, the answer is rounded up to 27 nights. Twenty-six nights would not give Sarah enough time.

17. D: This problem can be solved by using unit conversion. The initial units are miles per minute. The final units need to be feet per second. Converting miles to feet uses the equivalence statement 1 mile = 5,280 feet. Converting minutes to seconds uses the equivalence statement 1 minute = 60 seconds. Setting up the ratios to convert the units is shown in the following equation $\frac{72\ miles}{90\ minutes} * \frac{1\ minute}{60\ seconds} * \frac{5280\ feet}{1\ mile} = 70.4$ feet per second. The initial units cancel out, and the new units are left.

18. C: The sum total percentage of a pie chart must equal 100%. Since the CD sales take up less than half of the chart and more than a quarter (25%), it can be determined to be 40% overall. This can also be measured with a protractor. The angle of a circle is 360°. Since 25% of 360 would be 90° and 50% would be 180°, the angle percentage of CD sales falls in between; therefore, it would be Choice *C*.

19. B: Since $850 is the price *after* a 20% discount, $850 represents 80% of the original price. To determine the original price, set up a proportion with the ratio of the sale price (850) to original price (unknown) equal to the ratio of sale percentage:

$$\frac{850}{x} = \frac{80}{100}$$

(where *x* represents the unknown original price)

To solve a proportion, cross multiply the numerators and denominators and set the products equal to each other: (850) x (100) = (80) x (x). Multiplying each side results in the equation 85,000 = 80x.

To solve for *x*, both sides get divided by 80: $\frac{85,000}{80} = \frac{80x}{80}$, resulting in *x* = 1062.5. Remember that *x* represents the original price. Subtracting the sale price from the original price ($1062.50 – $850) indicates that Frank saved $212.50.

20. C: The decimal points are lined up, with zeroes put in as needed. Then, the numbers are added just like integers:

$$
\begin{array}{r}
3.40 \\
2.35 \\
+4.00 \\
\hline
9.75
\end{array}
$$

21. A: This problem can be multiplied as 588×32, except at the end, the decimal point needs to be moved three places to the left. Performing the multiplication will give 18,816, and moving the decimal place over three places results in 18.816.

22. D: The fraction is converted so that the denominator is 100 by multiplying the numerator and denominator by 4, to get $\frac{3}{25} = \frac{12}{100}$. Dividing a number by 100 just moves the decimal point two places to the left, with a result of 0.12.

23. A: Figure out which is largest by looking at the first non-zero digits. Choice B's first non-zero digit is in the hundredths place. The other three all have non-zero digits in the tenths place, so it must be A, C, or D. Of these, A has the largest first non-zero digit.

24. C: $40N$ would be 4000% of N. It's possible to check that each of the others is actually 40% of N.

25. B: Instead of multiplying these out, the product can be estimated by using $18 \times 10 = 180$. The error here should be lower than 15, since it is rounded to the nearest integer, and the numbers add to something less than 30.

26. C: 85% of a number means multiplying that number by 0.85. So, $0.85 \times 20 = \frac{85}{100} \times \frac{20}{1}$, which can be simplified to $\frac{17}{20} \times \frac{20}{1} = 17$.

27. A: To find the fraction of the bill that the first three people pay, the fractions need to be added, which means finding common denominator. The common denominator will be 60. $\frac{1}{5} + \frac{1}{4} + \frac{1}{3} = \frac{12}{60} + \frac{15}{60} + \frac{20}{60} = \frac{47}{60}$. The remainder of the bill is $1 - \frac{47}{60} = \frac{60}{60} - \frac{47}{60} = \frac{13}{60}$.

28. B: 30% is 3/10. The number itself must be 10/3 of 6, or $\frac{10}{3} \times 6 = 10 \times 2 = 20$.

29. A: First, these numbers should be converted to improper fractions: $\frac{7}{3} - \frac{11}{5}$. Take 15 as a common denominator: $\frac{7}{3} - \frac{11}{5} = \frac{35}{15} - \frac{33}{15} = \frac{2}{15}$.

30. B: Dividing by 98 can be approximated by dividing by 100, which would mean shifting the decimal point of the numerator to the left by 2. The result is 4.2 and rounds to 4.

31. B: $4\frac{1}{3} + 3\frac{3}{4} = 4 + 3 + \frac{1}{3} + \frac{3}{4} = 7 + \frac{1}{3} + \frac{3}{4}$. Adding the fractions gives $\frac{1}{3} + \frac{3}{4} = \frac{4}{12} + \frac{9}{12} = \frac{13}{12} = 1 + \frac{1}{12}$. Thus, $7 + \frac{1}{3} + \frac{3}{4} = 7 + 1 + \frac{1}{12} = 8\frac{1}{12}$.

32. C: The average is calculated by adding all six numbers, then dividing by 6. The first five numbers have a sum of 25. If the total divided by 6 is equal to 6, then the total itself must be 36. The sixth number must be 36 − 25 = 11.

33. B: Multiplying by 10^{-3} means moving the decimal point three places to the left, putting in zeroes as necessary.

34. B: $\frac{5}{2} \div \frac{1}{3} = \frac{5}{2} \times \frac{3}{1} = \frac{15}{2} = 7.5$.

35. A: The total fraction taken up by green and red shirts will be $\frac{1}{3}+\frac{2}{5}=\frac{5}{15}+\frac{6}{15}=\frac{11}{15}$. The remaining fraction is $1-\frac{11}{15}=\frac{15}{15}-\frac{11}{15}=\frac{4}{15}$.

36. C: If she has used 1/3 of the paint, she has 2/3 remaining. $2\frac{1}{2}$ gallons are the same as $\frac{5}{2}$ gallons. The calculation is $\frac{2}{3}\times\frac{5}{2}=\frac{5}{3}=1\frac{2}{3}$ gallons.

37. D: The correct answer of 20 °C can be found using the appropriate temperature conversion formula:

$$°C = (°F - 32) \times \frac{5}{9}$$

38. A: 12.018

Set up the problem, with the larger number on top and numbers lined up at the decimal. Place a zero at the end of the number with fewer digits to the right of the decimal (4.33 → 4.330), which does not change its value but makes for easier addition. Add, carrying anything over 9 into the next column to the left. Solve from right to left.

39. C: 29/36

Set up the problem and find a common denominator for both fractions.

$$\frac{7}{12}+\frac{2}{9}$$

Multiply each fraction across by the equivalent of 1 to convert to a common denominator.

$$\frac{7}{12}\times\frac{3}{3}+\frac{2}{9}\times\frac{4}{4}$$

Once over the same denominator, add across the top. The total is over the common denominator.

$$\frac{21+8}{36}=\frac{29}{36}$$

40. A: 18.853

Set up the problem, larger number on top and numbers lined up at the decimal. Begin subtracting with the far right column. Borrow 10 from the column to the left, when necessary.

41. B: 318.64

Set up the problem, with the larger number on top and numbers lined up at the decimal. Insert 0 in any blank spots to the right of the decimal as placeholders. Begin subtracting with the far right column. Borrow 10 from the column to the left, when necessary.

42. D: 1/3

Set up the problem and find a common denominator for both fractions.

$$\frac{39}{45}-\frac{8}{15}$$

Multiply each fraction across by 1 to convert to a common denominator.

$$\frac{39}{45} \times \frac{1}{1} - \frac{8}{15} \times \frac{3}{3}$$

Once over the same denominator, subtract across the top.

$$\frac{39 - 24}{45} = \frac{15}{45}$$

Reduce.

$$\frac{15 \div 15}{45 \div 15} = \frac{1}{3}$$

43. B: 4.11

Set up the problem, with the larger number on top. Multiply as if there are no decimal places. Add the answer rows together. Count the number of decimal places that were in the original numbers ($1 + 1 = 2$).

Place the decimal 2 places the right for the final solution.

44. B: 98.91

Set up the problem, with the larger number on top. Multiply as if there are no decimal places. Add the answer rows together. Count the number of decimal places that were in the original numbers (2).

Place the decimal in that many spots from the right for the final solution.

45. A: 20/63

Line up the fractions.

$$\frac{15}{21} \times \frac{48}{108}$$

Reduce the fractions prior to multiplying.

$$\frac{15 \div 3}{21 \div 3} = \frac{5}{7}$$

$$\frac{48 \div 4}{108 \div 4} = \frac{12}{27}$$

Multiply across the top and across the bottom.

$$\frac{5 \times 12}{7 \times 27} = \frac{60}{189}$$

Reduce.

$$\frac{60 \div 3}{189 \div 3} = \frac{20}{63}$$

46. D: $32\frac{19}{34}$

Set up the division problem.

$$34\overline{)1107}$$

44 does not go into 1 or 11 but will go into 110 so start there.

$$
\begin{array}{r}
32 \\
34\overline{)1107} \\
-102 \\
\hline
87 \\
-68 \\
\hline
19
\end{array}
$$

The answer is 32 19/34.

47. C: 9/46

Set up the division problem.

$$\frac{14}{28} \div \frac{23}{9}$$

Flip the second fraction and multiply.

$$\frac{14}{28} \times \frac{9}{23}$$

Simplify and reduce with cross multiplication.

$$\frac{1}{2} \times \frac{9}{23}$$

Multiply across the top and across the bottom.

$$\frac{1 \times 9}{2 \times 23} = \frac{9}{46}$$

48. A: 4 7/12

Divide.

$$12\overline{)55} \\ \underline{-48} \\ \ 7$$

The result is 4 7/12.

This cannot be reduced.

49. B: 59/6

The original number was 9 5/9. Multiply the denominator by the whole number portion. Add the numerator and put the total over the original denominator.

$$\frac{(6 \times 9) + 5}{6} = \frac{59}{6}$$

50. C: 2,718.035

To round 2,718.0354 to the nearest thousandths, use the digit in the ten-thousandths.

4 is less than 5, so round down in the thousandths.

2,718.035

Reading Comprehension

1. B: *A* is incorrect because it does not fit with the primary purpose of this passage, which is to tell a story of how a child plans to treat his parents when he sees the way they treat his grandfather. It is trying to remind readers to treat others with respect because that is how one wants to be treated, and that this does not apply only to elderly people. Choice *B* fits most appropriately with the primary purpose, since the son and wife see that they will be treated unfairly because they witness that their child plans to do it to them when they are older. To "reap what you sow" means that there are repercussions for every action. This may seem like the correct answer; however, the parents do not actually have to eat out of a trough later in life. They don't actually experience any repercussions. Even though it may be argued that the boy is being loyal to his grandfather, this does not fit with the primary purpose. The boy also never mentions that his actions are because he cares for his grandfather; rather, he simply mirrors the behaviors of his parents.

2. C: Although they do show him compassion in the end, it is not because they feel compassionate for him, but instead, it is because they recognize that their son plans to treat them the way they are treating the old man when they are older. So, they treat the old man the way they would want to be treated. Understanding is not the overall attitude they feel toward the old man, and it is only in realizing the cruelty of their behavior that they understand how they have been treating him. Choice *C* is correct because it condenses the actions of the son and his wife into a single word. Refusing to let the old man sit at the table when he clearly needs help and looks at the table with tear-filled eyes is a cruel thing to do. Choice *D* may be tempting to pick as they *are* impatient with him, but it's not the best answer. People can be impatient without being cruel.

3. D: They allow the old man to sit at the table because their son starts to make them a trough, so their motivation in letting him eat at the table is not because they feel sorry for him, but because they don't want their son to treat them that way when they are old. This makes Choice *A* incorrect. Their son did not tell them to let the old man sit at the table, so Choice *B* is incorrect. In the story, it mentions that even after the old man has eyes full of tears, the wife gave him a cheap wooden bowl to eat out of, so clearly his crying did not make them stop treating him badly, making Choice *C* incorrect. Choice *D* is correct because the parents let the old man sit at the table as a result of the boy mimicking their behavior.

4. C: Their name is more respected than the Danglars'. This inference question can be answered by eliminating incorrect answers. Choice *A* is tempting, considering that Albert mentions money as a concern in his marriage. However, although he may not be as rich as his fiancée, his father still has a stable income of 50,000 francs a year. Choice *B* isn't mentioned at all in the passage, so it's impossible to make an inference. Finally, Choice *D* is clearly false because Albert's father arranged his marriage but his mother doesn't approve of it. Evidence for Choice *C* can be found in the Count's comparison of Albert and Eugénie: "she will enrich you, and you will ennoble her." In other words, the Danglars are wealthier but the Morcef family has a more noble background.

5. D: Apprehensive. As in question 7, there are many clues in the passage that indicate Albert's attitude towards his marriage—far from enthusiastic, he has many reservations. This question requires test takers to understand the vocabulary in the answer choices. "Pragmatic" is closest in meaning to "realistic," and "indifferent" means "uninterested." The only word related to feeling worried, uncertain, or unfavorable about the future is "apprehensive."

6. B: He is like a wise uncle, giving practical advice to Albert. Choice *A* is incorrect because the Count's tone is friendly and conversational. Choice *C* is also incorrect because the Count questions why Albert doesn't want to marry a young, beautiful, and rich girl. While the Count asks many questions, he isn't particularly "probing" or "suspicious"—instead, he's asking to find out more about Albert's situation and then give him advice about marriage.

7. A: She belongs to a noble family. Though Albert's mother doesn't appear in the scene, there's more than enough information to answer this question. More than once is his family's noble background mentioned (not to mention that Albert's mother is the Comtess de Morcef, a noble title). The other answer choices can be eliminated—she is obviously deeply concerned about her son's future; money isn't her highest priority because otherwise she would favor a marriage with the wealthy Danglars; and Albert describes her "clear and penetrating judgment," meaning she makes good decisions.

8. C: The richest people in society were also the most respected. The Danglars family is wealthier but the Morcef family has a more aristocratic name, which gives them a higher social standing. Evidence for the other answer choices can be found throughout the passage: Albert mentioned receiving money from his father's fortune after his marriage; Albert's father has arranged this marriage for him; and the Count speculates that Albert's mother disapproves of this marriage because Eugénie isn't from a noble background like the Morcef family, implying that she would prefer a match with a girl from aristocratic society.

9. A: He seems reluctant to marry Eugénie, despite her wealth and beauty. This is a reading comprehension question, and the answer can be found in the following lines: "'I confess,' observed

Monte Cristo, "that I have some difficulty in comprehending your objection to a young lady who is both rich and beautiful."' Choice *B* is the opposite (Albert's father is the one who insists on the marriage), Choice *C* incorrectly represents Albert's eagerness to marry, and Choice *D* describes a more positive attitude than Albert actually feels ("repugnance").

10. B: Choice *B* is correct because having very little drinking water on earth is a very good reason that one should limit their water usage so that the human population does not run out of drinking water and die out. People wasting water on superfluous things does not support the fact that we need to limit our water usage. It merely states that people are wasteful. Therefore, *A* is incorrect. Answer Choice *C* may be tempting, but it is not the correct one, as this article is not about reducing water usage in order to help those who don't have easy access to water, but about the fact that the planet is running out of drinking water. Choice *D* is incorrect because nowhere in the article does it state that only first world countries have access to drinking water.

11. C: The primary purpose is to present a problem (the planet is running out of water) with a solution (to reduce water waste), therefore the correct answer is *C.* Choice *A* is incorrect because the passage does not have a sequential timeline of events, and is therefore not in chronological order. It may be tempting to think the author compares and contrasts people who do not have access to drinking water to those who do, but that does not fit with the primary purpose of the article, which is to convince people to reduce their water usage. Thus, Choice *B* is incorrect. Choice *D* is incorrect because descriptions are not the primary content of this article. Remember that a descriptive writing style describes people, settings, or situations in great detail with many adjectives. While a descriptive writing voice may be used alongside a persuasive writing style, it is generally not the primary voice when trying to convince a reader to take a certain stance.

12. A: The article is first person because it uses the pronoun "we," meaning the author is included as well as the reader. The author never addresses the reader directly, so *B* is incorrect. The perspective does not contain any third person pronouns, so *C* is incorrect. Since the correct answer is A but not B, then the answer cannot be *D.*

13. A: If the assertion is that the earth does not have enough drinking water, then having abundant water stores that are not being reported would certainly challenge this assertion. Choice *B* is incorrect because even if much of the water we drink does come from rain, that means the human population would be dependent on rain in order to survive, which would more support the assertion than challenge it. Because the primary purpose of the passage is not to help those who cannot get water, then Choice *C* is not the correct answer. Even if Choice *D* were true, it does not dismiss the other ways in which people are wasteful with water, and is also not the point.

14. B: Choice *B* is correct because the article uses a lot of emotionally charged language and also suggests what needs to be done with the information provided. The article does not contain elements of a narrative, which include plot, setting, characters, and themes. Not only does the article lack these things, but it does not follow a timeline, which is a key element of a narrative voice. Thus, Choice *A* is incorrect. Choice *C* is incorrect because the article uses information in order to be persuasive, but the purpose is not solely to inform on the issue. Choice *D* is incorrect because the article is not written in primarily descriptive language.

15. C: Choice *C* is correct because people who waste water on lawns in the desert, or run a half-full dishwasher, or fill their personal pools are not taking into account how much water they are using because they get an unlimited supply, therefore they are taking it for granted. Choice *A* is incorrect because it is explicitly stated within the text: "running dishwashers that are only half full." Choice B is also explicitly stated: "meanwhile people in Africa are dying of thirst." While Choice D is implicitly stated within the whole article, it is not implicitly stated within the sentence.

16. B: Choice B is correct because the author uses this example in order to show people, through emotional appeal, that they take water for granted, because they get water freely from their faucets, while millions of people have to endure great hardships to get drinking water. Choice A does not pertain directly to the main idea of the article, nor does it pertain to the author's purpose. The main idea is that people should reduce their water usage, and the author's purpose is to persuade the reader to do so. A person walking for miles in intense heat does not align with the main point. Choice C is incorrect because the selection never mentions that water is only available in first world countries. Choice D is the author's purpose for the entire passage, but not the purpose for mentioning the difficulty in getting water for some of the population.

17. C: To be mindful means to be aware, so C is the best answer. Choice A may be a tempting answer, because if people are interested in the water they are using, they may be more aware of it, but this is not the best answer of the choices. Being amused by water does not make sense in this context, so Choice B is incorrect. Being accepting of the amounts of water they use is the opposite of what the author is trying to get the reader to do. Thus, Choice D is incorrect.

18. A: The primary purpose and the main idea are essentially the same thing, and the main idea is that people should reduce their water usage because there is not a lot of available drinking water on Earth. Choice B is a *reason* that people should reduce their water usage, but it is not the main idea. Choice C is a demonstration of how people are not aware of the amount of water they use, but again, not the main idea. Choice D is a suggestion for reducing water usage, but still not the main idea.

19. C: All the details in this paragraph suggest that Brookside is a great place to live, plus the last sentence states that it is an *idyllic neighborhood*, meaning it is perfect, happy, and blissful. Choices A and B are incorrect, because although they do contain specific details from the paragraph that support the main idea, they are not the main idea. Choice D is incorrect because there is no reference in the paragraph to the crime rate in Brookside.

20. B: A passage like this one would likely appear in some sort of community profile, highlighting the benefits of living or working there. Choice A is incorrect because nothing in this passage suggests that it is fictional. It reads as non-fiction, if anything. Choice C is incorrect because it does not report anything particularly newsworthy, and Choice D is incorrect because it has absolutely nothing to do with a movie review.

21. D: In the first sentence, it states very clearly that the Brookside neighborhood is *one of the nation's first planned communities*. This makes it unique, as many other neighborhoods are old, many other neighborhoods exist in Kansas City, and many other neighborhoods have shopping areas. For these reasons, all the other answer choices are incorrect.

22. B: The author clearly states that education is crucial to the survival of the human race, and it can be easily inferred that if this is true, then improvements to our educational system are certainly worth fighting for. Choices A and C are incorrect because there is nothing in the passage that relates to these statements. Choice D is incorrect because it directly contradicts what the author states about all children's ability to learn.

23. A: Clearly, this author feels passionately about the importance of education. This is evident especially in the word choices. For this reason, all the other answer choices are incorrect.

24. C: Based on the author's passionate stance about the importance of education for all children, this answer choice makes the most sense. For this reason, all the other answer choices are incorrect.

25. D: The author mentions the importance of parent involvement and communication between school and home. He also devotes one full paragraph to the impact of technology on education. Nowhere in the passage does the author mention the cost of textbooks, so Choice *D* is correct.

21. D: *Enterprise* most closely means *cause*. Choices *A*, *B*, and *C* are all related to the term *enterprise*. However, Dickens speaks of a *cause* here, not a company, courage, or a game. *He will stand by such an enterprise* is a call to stand by a cause to enable the working man to have a certain autonomy over his own economic standing. The very first paragraph ends with the statement that the working man *shall . . . have a share in the management of an institution which is designed for his benefit.*

26. B: The speaker's salutation is one from an entertainer to his audience and uses the friendly language to connect to his audience before a serious speech. Recall in the first paragraph that the speaker is there to "accompany [the audience] . . . through one of my little Christmas books," making him an author there to entertain the crowd with his own writing. The speech preceding the reading is the passage itself, and, as the tone indicates, a serious speech addressing the "working man." Although the passage speaks of employers and employees, the speaker himself is not an employer of the audience, so Choice *A* is incorrect. Choice *C* is also incorrect, as the salutation is not used ironically, but sincerely, as the speech addresses the wellbeing of the crowd. Choice *D* is incorrect because the speech is not given by a politician, but by a writer.

28. B: For the working man to have a say in his institution which is designed for his benefit. Choice *A* is incorrect because that is the speaker's *first* desire, not his second. Choices *C* and *D* are tricky because the language of both of these is mentioned after the word *second*. However, the speaker doesn't get to the second wish until the next sentence. Choices *C* and *D* are merely prepositions preparing for the statement of the main clause, Choice *B*.

29. D: This is the correct answer choice because expository writing involves straightforward, factual information and analysis. It is unbiased and does not rely on the writer's personal feelings or opinions. Choice *A* is incorrect because narrative writing tells a story. Choice *B* is incorrect because persuasive writing is intended to change the reader's mind or position on a topic. Choice *C* is incorrect because technical writing attempts to outline a complex object or process.

30. B: This is the correct answer choice because the passage begins by describing Carver's childhood fascination with painting and later returns to this point when it states that at the end of his career "Carver returned to his first love of art." For this reason, all the other answer choices are incorrect.

31. A: This is the correct answer choice because the passage contains a definition of the term, *agricultural monoculture*, which is very similar to this answer.

32. C: This is the correct answer choice because there is ample evidence in the passage that refers to Carver's brilliance and the fact that his discoveries had a far-reaching impact both then and now. There is no evidence in the passage to support any of the other answer choices.

33. A: It introduces certain insects that transition from water to air. Choice *B* is incorrect because although the passage talks about gills, it is not the central idea of the passage. Choices *C* and *D* are incorrect because the passage does not "define" or "invite," but only serves as an introduction to stoneflies, dragonflies, and mayflies and their transition from water to air.

34. C: The act of shedding part or all of the outer shell. Choices *A*, *B*, and *D* are incorrect.

35. B: The first paragraph serves as a contrast to the second. Notice how the first paragraph goes into detail describing how insects are able to breathe air. The second paragraph acts as a contrast to the first by stating "[i]t is of great interest to find that, nevertheless, a number of insects spend much of their time under water." Watch for transition words such as "nevertheless" to help find what type of passage you're dealing with.

36: C: The stage of preparation in between molting is acted out in the water, while the last stage is in the air. Choices *A, B,* and *D* are all incorrect. *Instars* is the phase between two periods of molting, and the text explains when these transitions occur.

37. C: The author's tone is informative and exhibits interest in the subject of the study. Overall, the author presents us with information on the subject. One moment where personal interest is depicted is when the author states, "It is of great interest to find that, nevertheless, a number of insects spend much of their time under water."

38. C: This passage is designed to *persuade*. The whole purpose of the passage is to convince vacationers to come to Random Lake. There are some informative aspects of the passage, such as what's available – boating, house rentals, pontoon boats, but an extremely positive spin is put on the area, a spin that's designed to attract visitors. To prove it's persuasive, the argument can be reversed: Random Lake is *not* a good place to vacation. With a lack of adjectives and adverbs, there's a lack of *descriptive* detail, and this passage doesn't delight or *entertain* like a witty narrative might.

39. C: "Pontoon boats, kayaks, and paddle boats are available for rental" is out of place. The sentence before refers to fully furnished homes, and the sentence after refers to new developments. This sentence would have fit much better near, "Swimming, kayaking, boating, fishing, volleyball, mini-golf, go-cart track, eagle watching, nature trails," because the activities of the area are described. "This summer, why not rent a house on Random Lake?" is followed, logically, by a description of where Random Lake is. "There are enough activities there to keep a family busy for a month," is preceded by a listing of all those activities. "With several new housing developments slated for grand opening in March, the choices are endless!" links to "furnished houses," because this is an opportunity to find even more houses.

40. C: *The Random Lake area is growing.* This can be deduced with the passage, "With the Legends and The Broadmoor developments slated for grand openings in March, the choices are endless!" Considering buildings are being added, not razed, the Random Lake area would have to be growing. *Random City is more populated than Random Lake.* The word *city* is not necessarily indicative of size. There's simply not enough information to determine the size of either Random City or Random Lake. *The Random Lake area is newer than Random City.* Though this might seem logical with the addition of new buildings at Random Lake, there's no way to confirm this. The reader simply doesn't know enough about Random City to draw a comparison. *Random Lake prefers families to couples.* The ad definitely appeals to families but, "There are hotels available for every lifestyle and budget," proves that Random Lake is trying to appeal to everyone. Furthermore, "Prefer quiet? Historical? Modern?" proves that there are accommodations for every lifestyle.

41. A: The tone is exasperated. While contemplative is an option because of the inquisitive nature of the text, Choice *A* is correct because the speaker is annoyed by the thought of being included when he felt that the fellow members of his race were being excluded. The speaker is not nonchalant, nor accepting of the circumstances which he describes.

42. C: Choice *C*, *contented*, is the only word that has a different meaning. Furthermore, the speaker expresses objection and disdain throughout the entire text.

43. B: To address the feelings of exclusion expressed by African Americans after the establishment of the Fourth of July holiday. While the speaker makes biblical references, it is not the main focus of the passage, thus eliminating Choice *A* as an answer. The passage also makes no mention of wealthy landowners and doesn't speak of any positive response to the historical events, so Choices *C* and *D* are not correct.

44. D: Choice *D* is the correct answer because it clearly makes reference to justice being denied.

45. D: Hyperbole. Choices *A* and *B* are unrelated. Assonance is the repetition of sounds and commonly occurs in poetry. Parallelism refers to two statements that correlate in some manner. Choice *C* is incorrect because amplification normally refers to clarification of meaning by broadening the sentence structure, while hyperbole refers to a phrase or statement that is being exaggerated.

46. C: Throughout the entire text, the author maintains a persuasive tone. He argues that punishment should quickly follow the crime and gives a host of reasons why: it's more humane; it helps the prisoner to understand the nature of his or her crimes; it makes a better example for society. To confirm it's a persuasive stance, try reversing the argument. If the position cannot be reversed, then it's not persuasive. In this instance, the reader could argue in rebuttal that the punishment does not have to quickly follow the crime. Regardless of the veracity of this argument, simply creating it proves that the passage is persuasive.

47. C: This passage was written with a cause/effect structure. The cause is that the length between incarceration and trial should be as short as possible. The author, then, lists multiple effects of this cause. There are several key words that indicate this is a cause/effect argument. For instance, the author states, "The degree of the punishment, and the consequences of a crime, ought to be so contrived, as to have the greatest possible effect on others, with the least possible pain to the delinquent." The key words *as to have* indicate that changing the manner of punishment will change the outcome. Similarly, the authors states, "An immediate punishment is more useful; because the smaller the interval of time between the punishment and the crime, the stronger and more lasting will be the association of the two ideas of Crime and Punishment." Similar to *as to have* in the previous excerpt, *because* shows causation. In this instance, the author argues that the shorter the duration between crime and punishment, the more criminals will grasp the consequences of their actions. In general, for cause-effect passages, keep a lookout for words like *because*, *since*, *consequently*, *so*, and *as a result*.

48. D: "The more immediately after the commission of a crime a punishment is inflicted, the more just and useful it will be," best exemplifies the main idea of this passage. All subsequent discussion links back to this main idea and plays the role of supporting details. "The vulgar, that is, all men who have no general ideas or universal principles, act in consequence of the most immediate and familiar associations," supports this idea because the "vulgar," criminals, in other words, are used to making quick associations and are not used to delaying gratification or ignoring their impulses. "Crimes of less importance are commonly punished, either in the obscurity of a prison, or the criminal is transported, to give, by his slavery, an example to societies which he never offended," supports the main idea because the author argues that this is the wrong way to punish because if the punishment occurs in the same area the crime was committed, then the punishment will have more effect, since criminals will associate the areas with their crimes. Furthermore, transferring a prisoner takes time and delays punishment. Lastly, the author states, "Men do not, in general, commit great crimes deliberately, but rather in a sudden gust of passion; and they commonly look on the punishment due to a great crime as remote and improbable." To reduce the sense of punishments being remote and improbable, criminals must, according to the author, receive an immediate punishment. Therefore, by removing a lengthy gap between crime and punishment, a criminal's punishment will be close and probable, which the author argues is the most humane way to punish and the mark of a civilized society.

49. A: The author would disagree most strongly with the statement *criminals are incapable of connecting crime and punishment*. Though the author states that criminals are often passionate and consider punishment unlikely in the heat of the crime, the entire premise of the passage is that reducing the time between crime and punishment increases the likelihood of an association. He also argues that if a society does this consistently, the probability that individuals will consider the consequences of their actions increases. *A punishment should quickly follow the crime* is a restatement of the main idea, supported by evidence throughout the passage. *Most criminals do not think about the consequences of their actions*. Though the author makes this clear, he goes on to say that, in general, reducing the time between crime and punishment will have the most positive effect on the prisoner and on society. *Where a criminal is being punished is just as important as when*. The author argues in the passage that a punishment should be immediate and near where the crime originally occurred.

Vocabulary

1. D: Denigrating. To *denigrate* is to disparage or belittle.

2. C: Flushed. *Ruddy* means red and flushed.

3. A: Deduce. To *deduce* is to draw a logical conclusion or to infer.

4. B: Untoward. Something *untoward* is inconvenient and unexpected.

5. C: Any disorder of the nervous system that includes involuntary, jerky movements. It usually affects distal musculature and the face.

6. D: Itchiness. The intense itchiness of pruritis may be caused by dry skin, allergies, pregnancy, or other causes.

7. B: Ipsilateral. *Bilateral* is on both sides and *contralateral* is on opposite sides.

8. A: Excessive sweating. Causes of diaphoresis are varied and can include anxiety, medication side effects, malaria, and diabetes.

9. B: Sexually-transmitted. Syphilis and chlamydia are examples of venereal diseases.

10. C: Abjure. To *abjure* is to solemnly renounce a claim, belief, stance etc.

11. C: Harmful. Something *deleterious* causes damage or harm.

12. D: Anhedonia. *Hedonism* is the pursuit of pleasure. *Anhedonia* is often a sign of depression.

13. B: Subtle differences. *Nuances* are shades or subtle differences, particularly in tone, expression, or sound.

14. B: Distal means "situated away from." *Proximal* structures are closer to the trunk.

15. D: Phlegmatic. *Egregious* means appalling or shockingly bad. *Insolent* means rude and disrespectful. Something i*mpervious* does not allow fluid to penetrate or pass through.

16. C: Exogenous. Exogenous agents arise from outside the body.

17. A: Outlook. The *prognosis* is the expected likely course of an illness or injury.

18. D: Cachexia. *Catatonia* may occur with schizophrenia or other disorders and refers to an abnormality of behavior or movement. *Anorexia* refers to a loss of appetite or reduction of eating; it is often heard in association with the eating disorder anorexia nervosa. *Ataxia* refers to a loss of being able to fully control one's body parts.

19. C: To physically examine using touch. Medical professionals use their hands to palpate and feel an area of a patient's body to examine the physical structures using touch. They might detect lumps, areas of abnormal swelling, nodules, or other abnormalities.

20. D: Ancillary. Something *auxiliary* is ancillary or provides additional help or support. *Axillary* refers to the armpit.

21. A: Guileless. *Guileless* is to be without guile or deception, or to be innocent and childlike.

22. A: Inane. Someone described as *vacuous* lacks intelligence or thought. Something *vacuous* is inane or silly.

23. B: Dignity. *Gravitas* is dignity or seriousness of manner.

24. A: Adhesions. To *adhere* is to stick together, so adhesions are tissues sticking together.

25. C: Relating to the liver. The prefix *hepa-* relates to the liver.

26. D: The serous membrane lining the abdominal cavity. Choice *A* is referring to peristalsis. Choice *B* is referring to the perineum. Choice *C* is referring to the periosteum.

27. A: Ardent. *Vehement* means showing passionate feelings or being forceful.

28. A: Lumen. Arteries, blood vessels, and hollow organs have lumens.

29. C: Befuddled. *Lucid* means intelligible or expressed clearly, and *diffident* means modest or shy.

30. A: Decubitus ulcer. Bed sores are pressure ulcers or decubitus ulcers. They often occur in skin areas with underlying bony prominences, such as the heel or tailbone.

31. D: Afferent. Afferent nerves, for example, go from a receptor on the skin or other area of the body to the spinal cord. They relay sensory messages.

32. C: Dark scab. An eschar may result from a bad burn or from a mite bite or other causes.

33. C: Wan. *Pallor* means pale, lacking in color, or wan.

34. A: Nasal discharge. The prefix *rhin-* means nose or related to the nose, while the suffix *-rrhea* means flow or discharge. Menorrhea, for example, is menstrual flow.

35. B: Around the spinal cord. Baclofen, for spastic cerebral palsy, may have an intrathecal route of administration.

36. A: Verbally express grief. To *lament* is to mourn or verbally express sorrow or grief.

37. D: Harmful. Something noxious is poisonous, harmful, or very unpleasant.

38. C: An outward curvature of the thoracic spine. *Lordosis* is an exaggerated lumbar spine curve like swayback. *Scoliosis* is an abnormal lateral curvature of the spine.

39. D: The study of aging. The prefix *ger-* or *gero-* means old age as in geriatric.

40. B: Peptic ulcer. An endoscopy is a procedure that uses a flexible tube with a camera to visualize an internal structure.

41. B: Intransigent. *Complacent* means smug or self-satisfied. Something *inexplicable* cannot be accounted for or explained. *Confound* can mean to amaze or astonish, or to mix-up and cause difficulty distinguishing something.

42. B: Objective data. In SOAP notes, observable tests like blood pressure, weight, and pulse oximetry are recorded under the objective section.

43. A: One from which a patient will likely not recover. Examples of terminal illnesses are congestive heart failure, AIDs, and advanced kidney disease.

44. A: The knee. The shallow depression behind the knee is the popliteal fossa.

45. C: Paragon. A *parable* is like a fable or simple story, often with a moral lesson. A *paradox* is an apparent contradiction. *Paraphrase* can be a noun or a verb. As a noun, it is a rewording of something spoken or written, while as a verb, it means to use original language to reword what someone else wrote or said.

46. D: Clean and new. Something in pristine condition is unused or appears as it did when it was new.

47. A: Ringing in the ear. Tinnitus is a symptom of an underlying medical condition such as an ear injury or a circulation disturbance.

48. C: Inflammation. Tendonitis, conjunctivitis, and colitis are examples of medical conditions that are specific areas of inflammation.

49. C: Difficulty swallowing. The suffix *-phagia* usually refers to eating.

50. D: Hives. Urticaria may result from an allergic reaction to food, medicine, environmental trigger, or other allergen.

Grammar

1. A: The clause *that is autographed* is essential to the sentence so the word *that* is appropriate. *Whom* is the object of the verb *belongs to,* so you would not use *who.* Choice *B* is incorrect because the clause *which is autographed* is not enclosed in commas, and you would not use *who* as the object in the sentence. Choice *C* is incorrect because you would not use *whom* as the subject of the sentence and the clause *which is autographed* is not enclosed in commas. Choice *D* is incorrect because you would not use *whom* as the subject of the sentence.

2. A: The correct spelling of this word is *caffeine*. This answer, along with Choices *B* and *C* are exceptions to the rule *i before e, except after c*. Choice *D* follows this rule because the letters *ie* follow the letter *c*, so the correct order would be *ei*.

3. B: Use the word *may* instead of *can* at the beginning of the sentence because it is asking for permission and *can* means "able to." Choice *A* is a proper sentence using the word *bring* (coming toward) and the word *take* (going away) correctly. Choice *C* is a proper sentence using the word *lend* as a verb and the word *loan* as a noun. Choice *D* is a proper sentence using the words *two* (the number), *to* (the infinitive) and *too* (meaning "very") in the correct placements.

4. A: *Badly* is an adverb describing how hurt and *good* is used with the sensory word *feels*. Choice *B* is incorrect because *bad* is an adjective not an adverb. Choice *C* is incorrect because *bad* is an adjective where an adverb is needed and *well* is an adverb where an adjective is needed. Choice *D* is incorrect because *badly* fits but *good* should be used instead of *well* because of the sensory word *feels*.

5. C: *Because the lion and tiger habitat was closed* is a dependent clause and needs a subject. Choice *A* is incorrect because the sentence is an independent clause with both a subject and a verb, therefore it creates a complete sentence. Choice *B* is incorrect because the sentence is also a complete independent clause. Choice *D* is incorrect because the sentence is a complete independent clause forming an interrogative sentence.

6. A: *I love to go water-skiing, I love alpine skiing,* and *I also love Nordic skiing* are all independent clauses and are not connected with coordinating conjunctions or separated with semi colons, colons, or dashes. This makes it a run-on sentence. Choice *B* is not a run-on sentence; it is a simple single independent clause. Choice *C* is incorrect; it is a complete independent clause with both a subject (*types of skiing*) and a verb (*require*). Choice *D* is incorrect. It contains two independent clauses but a semicolon correctly separates them, therefore it is a complete compound sentence.

7. B: *Eating a large meal* cannot modify the word *food*. The food is not eating the meal. Choice *A* does not contain a dangling modifier. *Eating a large meal* modifies the pronoun *I*. Choice *C* does not contain a dangling modifier. It contains an incorrect preposition. The sentence should say, "*After eating a large meal, I was too full.*" Choice *D* does not contain a dangling modifier. *Eating a large meal* correctly modifies the pronoun *I*. *I* ate the large meal.

8. C: The word *impossible* is an absolute adjective. Something cannot be more or less impossible than something else. So *most impossible* is a double comparison. Choice *A* is incorrect because *more attainable* is the correct comparative degree of the adjective *attainable*. Choice *B* is incorrect because *most excited* is the correct superlative degree of the adjective *excited*. Choice *D* is incorrect because *less fortunate* is the correct form of the lesser degree of comparison for the adjective *fortunate*.

9. D: The necklace is the subject of the sentence and is receiving the action (being given away by Anna). Choice *A* is incorrect. Anna, the subject of the sentence, is also performing, not receiving, the action (*giving*). Choice *B* is incorrect. Although the necklace is the subject of the sentence there is no one specified to be performing the action of giving the necklace away. Choice *C* is incorrect. Anna (the subject) is not receiving the action in the sentence; instead the necklace is receiving the action of being given away.

10. B: The verb *will have hoped* tells us that the action will be completed before a future moment. For example, *"By the time this test is finished, you will have provided 50 answers."* Choice *A* is incorrect because *hope* is the present tense showing that the action is happening now, as in, *"I hope you got the answer correct."* Choice *C* is incorrect because *hoped* is the past tense of the base word *hope*. It tells us that the action has already been completed. Choice *D* is incorrect because *will hope* is the future tense telling us that the action will not be completed until sometime in the future.

11. C: The words *didn't* and *nothing* are both negatives. The sentence actually means a positive: *"They did like something I said."* Choice *A* is incorrect because it is a proper sentence with a single negative, *couldn't*. Choice *B* is incorrect because it is a proper sentence without any negatives. Choice *D* is incorrect because it is actually a triple negative; the words *cannot*, *don't*, and *disapprove* are all negatives. The sentence actually means: *"I disapprove of that."*

12. D: *Pulling heavy rope* is the subject complement for the word *helps*. Choice *A* is incorrect because *heavy rope* is the object complement for the word *pulling*. Choice *B* is incorrect because *muscles* is the object complement for the word *strengthen*. Choice *C* is incorrect because *strengthen* is the object complement for the word *helps*.

13. A: The words *whether/or not* are correlative conjunctions joining together two parts of the sentence that are alternative to one another. Choice *B* is incorrect because the word *and* joins two nouns, *Amber* and *Amanda;* therefore it is a coordinate conjunction. Choice *C* is incorrect because the word *while* in the sentence connects the dependent clause *they sat in their car* with the independent clause *it was raining*. Therefore it is a subordinate conjunction. Choice *D* is incorrect in several ways; the word *but* is a coordinate conjunction used at the beginning of an incomplete sentence.

14. B: The word *well* at the beginning of the sentence is set apart from the rest of the sentence with a comma and is a mild interjection. Choice *A* is incorrect. The word *goodness* at the end of the sentence is a noun. It is the idea/state of being for the cookie. Choice *C* is incorrect. It is an interrogative sentence and all of the words in the sentence can be identified as other parts of speech. *Can't* is a contraction of the word cannot and it works with the word *see* as the verb in the sentence. The word *you* is a pronoun; the word *that* is an adjective modifying the word *cookie*; *cookie* is a noun; *is* is another verb; and *broken* is an adjective modifying the word *cookie*. Choice *D* is incorrect because the exclamation mark at the end of the sentence is not there to set apart an interjection. Rather, it is there to punctuate the exclamatory sentence.

15. C: *I* needs to be capitalized because it begins a sentence and the pronoun *I* is always capitalized. The word *mother* needs to be capitalized because it is naming the name of a relative. The title of the book *All the Light We Cannot See* needs capitalization except for the article *the*. *Martha* needs to be capitalized because it is a proper noun. The word *she* needs to be capitalized because it is in the beginning of a sentence inside quotations. Choice *A* is incorrect because *I* at the beginning of the sentence needs to be capitalized and the words *favorite*, *book,* and *said* do not need capitalization because they are not proper nouns. Choice *B* is incorrect because *Mother* needs to be capitalized as a relative's name. *Book* is a common noun and does not need to be capitalized. The word *the* in the title of the book does not need to be capitalized because it is an article. *Said* does not need to be capitalized because it does not begin the sentence, and the word *she* needs to be capitalized because it does begin a new sentence inside quotation marks. Choice *D* is incorrect because the title *ALL THE LIGHT WE CANNOT SEE* should not be in all caps; rather it should be italicized and the first letter of each word should capitalized except *the*. It should be: *All the Light We Cannot See.*

16. C: There needs to be a period after the letters of the abbreviation *P.M.* There needs to be a period after the abbreviation *Dr.* There needs to be a period at the end of the declarative sentence. Choice *A* is incorrect because the periods after *P.M.* are omitted as is the period after the abbreviation *Dr.* The period after the end of the declarative sentence is also omitted. Choice *B* is incorrect because there is no ending punctuation for the declarative sentence and the periods in the abbreviation *P.M.* are omitted. Choice *D* is incorrect because the period after the word *forgotten* is extraneous.

17. D: *"Didn't anybody take the garbage out?"* is an interrogative sentence requiring a question mark for end punctuation. Choice *A* is incorrect because, *"Can you please take the garbage out,"* is an imperative sentence requiring a period for end punctuation. Choice *B* is incorrect because, *"I wonder if anyone has taken the garbage out,"* is a declarative sentence requiring a period for end punctuation. Choice *C* is incorrect because, *"Miles asked Lisa if she'd taken the garbage out,"* is also a declarative sentence.

18. B: *"Yikes!"* is an interjection. *"That startled me!"* is an exclamatory sentence. Both are punctuated with an exclamation mark. Choice *A* is incorrect because, *"Can you eat more than one slice of pizza!"* is an interrogative sentence so the end punctuation should be a question mark. Choice *C* is incorrect because we do not use both a question mark and an exclamation mark on the same sentence. Choice *D* is incorrect because we should never use more than one exclamation point in a grammatically correct sentence.

19. B: *A humanitarian* is a phrase describing the noun *Mother Teresa*, therefore it gets commas on both sides. There is a comma after *said* because the remark that follows is a quotation. Choice *A* is incorrect because there are extraneous commas after the words *two* and *three*. There only needs to be commas between the items in the list. Choice *C* is incorrect because there is an extraneous comma after the word *been*. Choice *D* is incorrect because there should be a period after the word *food,* and the word *consequently* should start a new sentence. The comma after the word *consequently* would be correct. There would not need to be a comma between *stomachache* and *heartburn* because it is a list of only two items.

20. D: There is a colon at the end of the introduction, *"There are four people who are most important to me."* There are serial commas already in a list—*my husband, my daughter, my friend, and my sister*—separated by semicolons after the names of each person. Choice *A* is incorrect because there are only semicolons separating the introduction and the items in the list. Choice *B* is incorrect because there is an extraneous colon between *people* and *who* and because the items in the list are only separated by commas. Choice *C* is incorrect because a semicolon instead of a colon separates the introduction from the list, and colons instead of semicolons separate the names of the people. In other words, in choice *C* the roles of the colon and semicolon are reversed.

21. A: There should be a comma after the introduction *Daniel said* because it is a short quote. Quotation marks belong before and after exactly what was said, *"I want to travel to Mars,"* and the period belongs inside the quotation marks. Choice *B* is incorrect because there is no comma after the introduction, and the period is outside the quotation marks. Choice *C* is incorrect because the quotes are not around the actual statement, just the fragment *travel to Mars;* also, the period is outside the quotation marks. Choice *D* is incorrect because the quotations are enclosing the entire sentence, not just what was said, and there is no comma after the introduction.

22. C: The *team* is a collective noun acting as one, and therefore a singular verb *competes* creates subject/verb agreement. Choice *A* is incorrect. *Teams* is a plural subject, and *competes* is a singular verb; they do not create subject/verb agreement. Choice *B* is incorrect. *Teams* is plural, and *wins* is singular; they do not create subject/verb agreement. Choice *D* is incorrect. *Team* is a collective noun acting as one and agrees with a singular verb, but *win* is plural.

23. A: The *professor* is the singular subject (*of physics* should be ignored) and *compliments* is a singular verb. Choice *B* is incorrect. *Professor* is the singular subject but *compliment* is a plural verb. Choice *C* is incorrect. *Professors* is a plural subject and *compliments* is a singular verb; they do not agree. Choice *D* is incorrect; adding the word *will* to *compliments* does not change the fact that *compliments* is a singular verb and does not agree with the plural subject *professors*.

24. A: It is necessary to put a comma between the date and the year and between the day of the week and the month. Choice *B* is incorrect because it is missing the comma between the day of the week and the month. Choice *C* is incorrect because it adds an unnecessary comma between the month and date. Choice *D* is missing the necessary comma between day of the week and month.

25. B: *Conscientious* and *judgment* are both spelled correctly in this sentence. These are both considered commonly misspelled words. One or both words are spelled incorrectly in all the other examples.

26. B: In this sentence, the word *stress* is a noun. While the word *stress* can also act as a verb, in this particular case, it functions as a noun as the subject of the sentence. The word *stress* cannot be used as an adjective or adverb, so these answers are also incorrect.

27. B: The correct answer is o*ctopi,* the plural form of the word *octopus*. Choice *A* is the incorrect spelling of the plural of *roof*, which should be *roofs*. Choice *C* is the incorrect spelling of the plural form of the word *potato*, which should be *potatoes.* Choice *D* is the incorrect plural form of the word *fish*, which remains the same in the singular and the plural, *fish.*

28. A: Quotation marks are used to indicate something someone has said. This is a direct quotation that interrupts, or breaks, the sentence in half. A comma is necessary before the quotation and after it, and inside the quotation marks, to set off the quote from the rest of the sentence. Choice *B* is incorrect because there is no comma at the end of the quotation. Choice *C* is incorrect because there is no comma before or after the quotation. Choice *D* is incorrect because the comma at the end of the quotation is placed outside the quotation marks.

29. C: In this sentence, the word *counter* functions as an adjective that modifies the word *argument*. Choice *A* is incorrect because the word *counter* functions as a noun. Choice *B* is incorrect because the word *counter* functions as a verb. Choice *D* is incorrect because the word *counter* functions as an adverb.

30. B: This sentence correctly uses the plural pronoun *their,* which agrees in number with its antecedent, *human beings*. Choice *A* is incorrect because *his* is a singular pronoun and does not agree in number with the antecedent. Choice *C* is incorrect because *its* is a singular pronoun and usually refers to an object. Choice *D* is incorrect because *her* is a singular pronoun and does not agree with the antecedent.

31. D: *Every single one of my mother's siblings, their spouses, and their children* is the complete subject because it includes who or what is doing the action in the sentence as well as the modifiers that go with it. The other answer choices are incorrect because they only include part of the complete subject.

32. A: The word *foliage* is defined as leaves on plants or trees. In this sentence, the meaning can be drawn from the fact that a heavily wooded area in October would be characterized by the beautiful changing colors of the leaves. The other answer choices do not accurately define the word *foliage*, so they are incorrect.

33. C: Choice *C* is the one that incorrectly uses italics; quotation marks should be used for the title of a short work such as a poem, not italics. Choice *A* correctly italicizes the title of a novel. Choice *B* correctly italicizes the title of both musicals, and Choice *D* correctly italicizes the name of a work of art.

34. A: In this sentence, the commonly misused words *it's* and *than* are used correctly. *It's* is a contraction for the pronoun *it* and the verb *is*. The word *than* accurately shows comparison between two things. The other examples all contain some combination of the commonly misused words *then* and *its*. *Then* is an adverb that conveys time, and *its* is a possessive pronoun. Both are incorrectly used in the other examples.

35. C: This example is an imperative sentence because it gives a command and ends with a period. Choice *A* is a declarative sentence that states a fact and ends with a period. Choice *B* is an interrogative sentence that asks a question and ends with a question mark. Choice *D* is an exclamatory sentence that shows strong emotion and ends with an exclamation point.

36. D: This is a compound sentence because it joins two independent clauses, *Felix plays the guitar in my roommate's band* and *Alicia is the lead vocalist*, with a comma and the coordinating conjunction *and*. Choices *A* and *C* are simple sentences, each containing one independent clause with a complete subject and predicate. Choice *A* does contain a compound subject, *John and Adam,* and Choice *C* contains a compound predicate, *ran and went*, but they are still simple sentences that only contain one independent clause. Choice *B* is a complex sentence because it contains one dependent clause, *As I was leaving,* and one independent clause, *my dad called and needed to talk.* This sentence also contains a compound predicate*, called and needed.*

37. B: This answer includes all the words functioning as nouns in the sentence. Choice *A* is incorrect because it does not include the proper noun *Monday*. The word *he* makes Choice *C* incorrect because it is a pronoun. This example also includes the word *dorm*, which can function as a noun, but in this sentence, it functions as an adjective modifying the word *room*. Choice *D* is incorrect because it leaves out the proper noun *Jose*.

38. D: The simple subject of this sentence, *Everyone*, although it names a group, is a singular noun and therefore agrees with the singular verb form *has*. Choice *A* is incorrect because the simple subject *each* does not agree with the plural verb form *have*. In Choice *B*, the plural subject *players* does not agree with the singular verb form *was*. In Choice *C*, the plural subject *friends* does not agree with the singular verb form *has*.

39. A: In this sentence, the word *Mom* should not be capitalized because it is not functioning as a proper noun. If the possessive pronoun *My* was not there, then it would be considered a proper noun and would be capitalized. *East Coast* is correctly capitalized. Choice *B* correctly capitalizes the name of a specific college course, which is considered a proper noun. Choice *C* correctly capitalizes the name of a specific airline, which is a proper noun, and Choice *D* correctly capitalizes the proper nouns *Martha's Vineyard* and *New England*.

40. C: In this sentence, *exhilarating* is functioning as an adjective that modifies the word *morning*, which in turn, modifies the word *air*. The words *air* and *morning* are functioning as nouns, and the word *inspired* is functioning as a verb in this sentence. Other words functioning as adjectives in the sentence include, *beautiful, mountain, every,* and *lengthy.*

41. D: This is the correct answer because the pronouns *him* and *me* are in the objective case. *Him* and *me* are the indirect objects of the verb *gave.* Choice *A* is incorrect because the personal pronoun in this case, *me,* should always go last. Choices *B* and *C* are incorrect because they contain at least one subjective pronoun.

42. B: In this sentence, a colon is correctly used to introduce a series of items. Choice *A* incorrectly uses a semicolon to introduce the series of states. Choice *C* incorrectly uses a dash to introduce the series. Choice *D* is incorrect because it incorrectly uses a comma to introduce the series.

43. A: This sentence uses the correct form of the contraction *you are* as the subject of the sentence, and it uses the correct form of the possessive pronoun *your* to indicate ownership of the backpack. It also uses the correct form of the adverb *there,* indicating place and the possessive pronoun *their* indicating ownership. Choice *B* is incorrect because it reverses the possessive pronoun *your* and the contraction *you are.* Choice *C* is incorrect because it reverses the adverb *there* and the possessive pronoun *their.* Choice *D* is incorrect because it reverses the contraction *you are* and the possessive pronoun *your* and the possessive pronoun *their* and the adverb *there.*

44. A: In this sentence, the subject *car* is acted upon, rather than completing the action of the sentence. To put this sentence into active voice, the subject should be the hail. Example: *The hail during the storm the other night terribly dented my car.* All the other sentences use active voice because the subject is completing the action of the sentence.

45. C: This sentence correctly places an apostrophe after the plural proper noun *Joneses* to show possession. When a proper name ends in *s,* it is necessary to add *–es* to make it plural, then an apostrophe to make the plural form possessive. In Choice *A,* to make the word *children* possessive, add an apostrophe and then *-s* since the word *children* is already plural. Choice *B* does not need an apostrophe because *Smiths* is plural, not possessive. Choice *D* incorrectly places an apostrophe after the *–s.* In this case, to make *people* possessive, it is necessary to add an apostrophe and then an *–s* since the word *people* is already plural.

46. A: When parallel structure is used, all parts of the sentence are grammatically consistent. Choice *A* uses incorrect parallel structure because *swimming* and *biking* are gerunds, whereas *a run* is an infinitive, so the structure is grammatically inconsistent. Choices *B, C,* and *D* all have lists that are grammatically consistent.

47. C: The original sentence states that despite the author being nervous, she was able to read with poise and confidence, which is stated in Choice *C.* Choice *A* changes the meaning by adding *because;* however, the author didn't read with confidence *because* she was nervous, but *despite* being nervous. Choice *B* is closer to the original meaning; however, it loses the emphasis of her succeeding *despite* her condition. Choice *D* adds the word *before,* which doesn't make much sense on its own, much less in relation to the original sentence.

48. D: The original sentence states that there was a storm surge and loss of electricity during the hurricane, making Choice *D* correct. Choices *A* and *B* arrange the storm surge and the loss of electricity within a cause and effect statement, which changes the meaning of the original sentence. Choice *C* changes *surge* from a noun into a verb and creates an entirely different situation.

49. B: The original sentence states that an elephant herd will help and support another herd member if it is sick, so Choice *B* is correct. Choice *A* is incorrect because it states the whole herd will be too sick and too tired to walk instead of a single elephant. Choice *C* is incorrect because the original sentence does not say that the herd gathers food when *they* are sick, but when a single member of the herd is sick. Although Choice *D* might be correct in a general sense, it does not relate to the meaning of the original sentence and is therefore incorrect.

50. A: The original sentence says that after a soccer game, they went out to eat. Choice *A* shows the same sequence: they finished the soccer game *then* went out to eat. Choice *B* is incorrect because it reverses the sequence of events. Choices *C* and *D* are incorrect because the words *so* and *because* change the meaning of the original sentence.

Biology

1. C: Molecules that are soluble in lipids, like fats, sterols, and vitamins (A, D, E and K), for example, are able to move in and out of a cell using passive transport. Water and oxygen are also able to move in and out of the cell without the use of cellular energy. Complex sugars and non-lipid soluble molecules are too large to move through the cell membrane without relying on active transport mechanisms. Molecules naturally move from areas of high concentration to those of lower concentration. It requires active transport to move molecules in the opposite direction, as suggested by Choice *D*.

2. A: Both types of cells are enclosed by plasma membranes with cytosol on the inside. Prokaryotes contain a nucleoid and do not have organelles; eukaryotes contain a nucleus enclosed by a membrane, as well as organelles.

3. B: During telophase, two nuclei form at each end of the cell and nuclear envelopes begin to form around each nucleus. The nucleoli reappear, and the chromosomes become less compact. The microtubules are broken down by the cell, and mitosis is complete. The process begins with prophase as the mitotic spindles begin to form from centrosomes. Prometaphase follows, with the breakdown of the nuclear envelope and the further condensing of the chromosomes. Next, metaphase occurs when the microtubules are stretched across the cell and the chromosomes align at the metaphase plate. Finally, in the last step before telophase, anaphase occurs as the sister chromatids break apart and form chromosomes.

4. D: Meiosis has the same phases as mitosis, except that they occur twice—once in meiosis I and once in meiosis II. During meiosis I, the cell splits into two. Each cell contains two sets of chromosomes. Next, during meiosis II, the two intermediate daughter cells divide again, producing four total haploid cells that each contain one set of chromosomes.

5. D: DNA and RNA each contain four nitrogenous bases, three of which they have in common: adenine, guanine, and cytosine. Thymine is only found in DNA, and uracil is only found in RNA. Adenine interacts with uracil in RNA, and with thymine in DNA. Guanine always pairs with cytosine in both DNA and RNA.

6. B: Dominant alleles are considered to have stronger phenotypes and, when mixed with recessive alleles, will mask the recessive trait. The recessive trait would only appear as the phenotype when the allele combination is "aa" because a dominant allele is not present to mask it.

7. A: Speciation is the method by which one species splits into two or more species. In allopatric speciation, one population is divided into two subpopulations. If a drought occurs and a large lake becomes divided into two smaller lakes, each lake is left with its own population that cannot intermingle with the population of the other lake. When the genes of these two subpopulations are no longer mixing with each other, new mutations can arise and natural selection can take place.

8. C: In the Linnean system, organisms are classified as follows, moving from comprehensive and specific similarities to fewer and more general similarities: species, genus, family, order, class, phylum, kingdom, and domain. A popular mnemonic device to remember the Linnean system is "Dear King Philip came over for good soup."

9. A: Fungal cells have a cell wall, similar to plant cells; however, they use oxygen as a source of energy and cannot perform photosynthesis. Because they do not perform photosynthesis, fungal cells do not contain chloroplasts.

10. A: Roots are responsible for absorbing water and nutrients that will get transported up through the plant. They also anchor the plant to the ground. Photosynthesis occurs in leaves, stems transport materials through the plant and support the plant body, and phloem moves sugars downward to the leaves.

11. D: Tropism is a response to stimuli that causes the plant to grow toward or away from the stimuli. Hydrotropism is a response to a change in water concentration. Phototropism is a reaction to light that causes plants to grow toward the source of the light. Thermotropism is a response to changes in temperature. Gravitropism is a response to gravity that causes roots to follow the pull of gravity and grow downward, but also causes plant shoots to act against gravity and grow upward.

12. C: Population dynamics looks at the composition of populations, including size and age, and the biological and environmental processes that cause changes. These can include immigration, emigration, births, and deaths.

13. A: Ecosystems are maintained by cycling the energy and nutrients that they obtain from external sources. The process can be diagramed in a food web, which represents the feeding relationship between the species in a community. A phylogenetic tree shows inferred evolutionary relationships among species and is similar to the fossil record. A pedigree chart shows occurrences of phenotypes of a particular gene through the generations of an organism.

14. B: The endocrine system's organs are glands which are spread throughout the body. The endocrine system itself does not connect the organs or transport the hormones they secrete. Rather, the various glands secrete the hormone into the bloodstream and lets the cardiovascular system pump it throughout the body. The other three body systems each include a network throughout the body:

- Cardiovascular system: veins and arteries
- Immune system: lymphatic vessels (it does also use the circulatory system)
- Nervous system: nerve networks

15. D: In the secondary immune response, suppressor T lymphocytes are activated to negate the potential risk of damage to healthy cells, brought on by an unchecked, overactive immune response. Choice *A* is incorrect because the activity is characteristic of the primary response, not the secondary response Choice *B* is incorrect because humeral immunity is mediated by antibodies produced by B, not T, lymphocytes. Choice *C* is wrong because the secondary response is faster than the primary response because the primary response entails the time-consuming process of macrophage activation.

16. A: Keratin is a structural protein and it is the primary constituent of things like hair and nails. Choice *B* is incorrect antigens are immune proteins that help fight disease. Hormonal proteins are responsible for initiating the signal transduction cascade to regulate gene expression. Choice *C* is incorrect because channel proteins are transport proteins that help move molecules into and out of a cell. Marker proteins help identify or distinguish a cell. Lastly, Choice *D* is incorrect because actin, like myosin, is a motor protein because it is involved in the process of muscle contraction.

17. C: The lagging strand of DNA falls behind the leading strand because of its discontinuous synthesis. DNA helicase unzips the DNA helices so that synthesis can take place, and RNA primers are created by the RNA primase for the polymerases to attach to and build from. The lagging strand is synthesizing DNA in a direction that is hard for the polymerase to build, so multiple primers are laid down so that the entire length of DNA can be synthesized simultaneously, piecemeal. These short pieces of DNA being synthesized are known as Okazaki fragments and are joined together by DNA ligase.

18. D: Germline mutations in eggs and sperm are permanent, can be on the chromosomal level, and will be inherited by offspring. Somatic mutations cannot affect eggs and sperm, and therefore are not inherited by offspring. Mutations of either kind are rarely beneficial to the individual, but do not necessarily harm them. Germline cells divide much more rapidly than do somatic cells, and a mutation in a sex cell would promulgate and affect many thousands of its daughter cells.

19. B: Biological catalysts are termed *enzymes*, which are proteins with conformations that specifically manipulate reactants into positions which decrease the reaction's activation energy. Lipids do not usually affect reactions, and cofactors, while they can aid or be necessary to the proper functioning of enzymes, do not make up the majority of biological catalysts.

20. C: mRNA is directly transcribed from DNA before being taken to the cytoplasm and translated by rRNA into a protein. tRNA transfers amino acids from the cytoplasm to the rRNA for use in building these proteins. siRNA is a special type of RNA which interferes with other strands of mRNA typically by causing them to get degraded by the cell rather than translated into protein.

21. B: Since the genotype is a depiction of the specific alleles that an organism's genes code for, it includes recessive genes that may or may not be otherwise expressed. The genotype does not have to name the proteins that its alleles code for; indeed, some of them may be unknown. The phenotype is the physical, visual manifestations of a gene, not the genotype. The genotype does not necessarily include any information about the organism's physical characters. Although some information about an organism's parents can be obtained from its genotype, its genotype does not actually show the parents' phenotypes.

22. C: One in four offspring (or 25%) will be short, so all four offspring cannot be tall. Although both of the parents are tall, they are hybrid or heterozygous tall, not homozygous. The mother's phenotype is for tall, not short. A Punnett square cannot determine if a short allele will die out. Although it may seem intuitive that the short allele will be expressed by lower numbers of the population than the tall allele, it still appears in 75% of the offspring (although its effects are masked in 2/3 of those). Besides, conditions could favor the recessive allele and kill off the tall offspring.

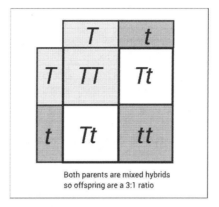

Both parents are mixed hybrids
so offspring are a 3:1 ratio

23. A: Human genes are strictly DNA and do not include proteins or amino acids. A human's genome and collection of genes will include even their recessive traits, mutations, and unused DNA.

24. C: To gather accurate data, the student must be able compare a participant's test score from round 1 with their test score from round 2. The differing levels of intellect among the participants means that comparing participants' test scores to those of other participants would be inaccurate. This requirement excludes choices A and D, which involve only one round of testing. The experiment must also involve different levels of sugar consumption from round 1 to round 2. In this way, the effects of different levels of sugar consumption can be seen on the same subjects. Thus, B is incorrect because the experiment provides for no variation of sugar consumption. C is the correct answer because it allows the student to compare each participant's test score from round 1 with their test score from round 2 after different level of sugar consumption.

25. D: *D* is the correct answer because excess sunlight is a common cause of plant wilting. *A*, *B*, and *C* are all possible but unlikely to be a cause for wilting. Given that the test question asks for a *reasonable* explanation, *sunlight* is by far the most reasonable answer.

Chemistry

1. D: Nuclear reactions take place in the nucleus of certain unstable atoms. They involve a change in the structure of the nucleus, through some type of decomposition, and energy is released. Unlike in regular chemical reactions where mass is conserved, in nuclear reactions, there is a change in mass between the reactants and products.

2. A: A Lewis Dot diagram shows the alignment of the valence (outer) shell electrons and how readily they can pair or bond with the valence shell electrons of other atoms to form a compound. Choice *B* is incorrect because the Lewis Dot structure aids in understanding how likely an atom is to bond or not bond with another atom, so the inner shell would add no relevance to understanding this likelihood. The positioning of protons and neutrons concerns the nucleus of the atom, which again would not lend information to the likelihood of bonding.

3. B: A decomposition reaction breaks down a compound into its constituent elemental components. Choice *A* is incorrect because a synthesis reaction joins two or more elements into a single compound. Choice *C*, an organic reaction, is not possible, since it needs carbon and hydrogen for a reaction. Choice *D*, oxidation/reduction (redox or half) reaction, is incorrect because it involves the loss of electrons from one species (oxidation) and the gain of electrons to the other species (reduction). There is no notation of this occurring within the given reaction, so it is incorrect.

4. C:

$$2Na + Cl_2 \longrightarrow 2NaCl$$

The number of each element must be equal on both sides of the equation:

Choice C is the only correct option: $2Na + Cl_2 \rightarrow 2NaCl$

2 Na + 2 Cl does equal 2 Na + 2 Cl (the number of sodium atoms and chlorine atoms match)

Choice A: $Na + Cl_2 \rightarrow NaCl$

1 Na + 2 Cl does not equal 1 Na + 1 Cl (the number of chlorine atoms do not match)

Choice B: $2Na + Cl_2 \rightarrow NaCl$

2 Na + 2 Cl does not equal 1 Na + 1 Cl (neither the number of sodium atoms nor chlorine atoms match)

Choice D: $2Na + 2Cl_2 \rightarrow 2NaCl$

2 Na + 4 Cl does not equal 2 Na + 2 Cl (the number of chlorine atoms do not match)

5. D: The naming of compounds focuses on the second element in a chemical compound. Elements from the non-metal category are written with an "ide" at the end. The compound CO has one carbon and one oxygen, so it is called carbon monoxide. Choice B represents that there are two oxygen atoms, and Choices A and B incorrectly alter the name of the first element, which should remain as carbon.

6. B: To solve this, the number of moles of NaCl needs to be calculated:

First, to find the mass of NaCl, the mass of each of the molecule's atoms is added together as follows:

$$23.0g \text{ (Na)} + 35.5g \text{ (Cl)} = 58.8g \text{ NaCl}$$

Next, the given mass of the substance is multiplied by one mole per total mass of the substance:

$$4.0g \text{ NaCl} \times (1 \text{ mol NaCl}/58.5g \text{ NaCl}) = 0.068 \text{ mol NaCl}$$

Finally, the moles are divided by the number of liters of the solution to find the molarity:

$$(0.068 \text{ mol NaCl})/(0.120L) = 0.57 \text{ M NaCl}$$

Choice A incorporates a miscalculation for the molar mass of NaCl, and Choices C and D both incorporate a miscalculation by not converting mL into liters (L), so they are incorrect by a factor of 10.

7. C: According to the *ideal gas law* ($PV = nRT$), if volume is constant, the temperature is directly related to the pressure in a system. Therefore, if the pressure increases, the temperature will increase in direct proportion. Choice A would not be possible, since the system is closed and a change is occurring, so the temperature will change. Choice B incorrectly exhibits an inverse relationship between pressure and temperature, or $P = 1/T$. Choice D is incorrect because even without actual values for the variables, the relationship and proportions can be determined.

8. D: Density is found by dividing mass by volume:

$$density = \frac{mass}{volume}$$

The unit for mass (in this case grams) and the units for volume (in this case cm^3) need to be combined together. They're combined as grams over volume since that's how they were set up in the equation:

$$d = \frac{14.3\ g}{5.4\ cm^3} = 2.65\ g/cm^3$$

9. C: 2:9:10:4. These are the coefficients that follow the law of conservation of matter. The coefficient times the subscript of each element should be the same on both sides of the equation.

10. C: A catalyst functions to increase reaction rates by decreasing the activation energy required for a reaction to take place. Inhibitors would increase the activation energy or otherwise stop the reactants from reacting. Although increasing the temperature usually increases a reaction's rate, this is not true in all cases, and most catalysts do not function in this manner.

11. D: Mass refers to the amount or quantity there is of an object. Light, sound, and heat are all forms of energy that can travel in waves.

12. A: Salts are formed from compounds that use ionic bonds. Disulfide bridges are special bonds in protein synthesis which hold the protein in their secondary and tertiary structures. Covalent bonds are strong bonds formed through the sharing of electrons between atoms and are typically found in organic molecules like carbohydrates and lipids. London dispersion forces are fleeting, momentary bonds which occur between atoms that have instantaneous dipoles but quickly disintegrate.

13. C: As in the last question, covalent bonds are special because they share electrons between multiple atoms. Most covalent bonds are formed between the elements H, F, N, O, S, and C, while hydrogen bonds are formed nearly exclusively between H and either O, N, or F. Covalent bonds may inadvertently form dipoles, but this does not necessarily happen. With similarly electronegative atoms like carbon and hydrogen, dipoles do not form, for instance. Crystal solids are typically formed by substances with ionic bonds like the salts sodium iodide and potassium chloride.

14. A: Gases like air will move and expand to fill their container, so they are considered to have an indefinite shape and indefinite volume. Liquids like water will move and flow freely, so their shapes change constantly, but do not change volume or density on their own. Solids change neither shape nor volume without external forces acting on them, so they have definite shapes and volumes.

15. D: Evaporation takes place at the surface of a fluid while boiling takes place throughout the fluid. The liquid will boil when it reaches its boiling or vaporization temperature, but evaporation can happen due to a liquid's volatility. Volatile substances often coexist as a liquid and as a gas, depending on the pressure forced on them. The phase change from gas to liquid is condensation, and both evaporation and boiling take place in nature.

16. C: Water's polarity lends it to be extremely cohesive and adhesive; this cohesion keeps its atoms very close together. Because of this, it takes a large amount of energy to melt and boil its solid and liquid forms. Phospholipid bilayers are made of nonpolar lipids and water, a polar liquid, cannot flow through it. Cell membranes use proteins called aquaporins to solve this issue and let water flow in and out. Fish breathe by capturing dissolved oxygen through their gills. Water can self-ionize, wherein it decomposes into a hydrogen ion (H⁺) and a hydroxide ion (OH⁻), but it cannot self-hydrolyze.

17. D: An isotope of an element has an atomic number equal to its number of protons, but a different mass number because of the additional neutrons. Even though there are differences in the nucleus, the behavior and properties of isotopes of a given element are identical. Atoms with different atomic numbers also have different numbers of protons and are different elements, so they cannot be isotopes.

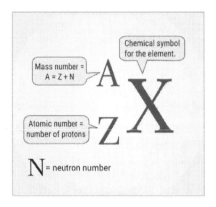

18. A: The neutrons and protons make up the nucleus of the atom. The nucleus is positively charged due to the presence of the protons. The negatively charged electrons are attracted to the positively charged nucleus by the electrostatic or Coulomb force; however, the electrons are not contained in the nucleus. The positively charged protons create the positive charge in the nucleus, and the neutrons are electrically neutral, so they have no effect. Radioactivity does not directly have a bearing on the charge of the nucleus.

19. C: Neon, one of the noble gases, is chemically inert or not reactive because it contains eight valence electrons in the outermost shell. The atomic number is 10, with a 2.8 electron arrangement meaning that there are 2 electrons in the inner shell and the remaining 8 electrons in the outer shell. This is extremely stable for the atom, so it will not want to add or subtract any of its electrons and will not react under typical circumstances.

20. D: The law states that matter cannot be created or destroyed in a closed system. In this equation, there are the same number of molecules of each element on either side of the equation. Matter is not gained or lost, although a new compound is formed. As there are no ions on either side of the equation, no electrons are lost. The law prevents the hydrogen from losing mass and prevents oxygen atoms from being spontaneously spawned.

21. B: A solid produced during a reaction is called a *precipitate.* In a neutralization reaction, the products (an acid and a base) react to form a salt and water. Choice *A*, an oxidation reaction, involves the transfer of an electron. Choice *C*, a synthesis reaction, involves the joining of two molecules to form a single molecule. Choice *D*, a decomposition reaction, involves the separation of a molecule into two other molecules.

22. A: The decimal point for this value is located after the final zero. Because the decimal is moved 12 places to the left in order to get it between the *8* and the *6*, then the resulting exponent is positive, so Choice *A* is the correct answer. Choice *B* is false because the decimal has been moved in the wrong direction. Choice *C* is incorrect because the decimal has been moved an incorrect number of times. Choice *D* is false because this value is written to three significant figures, not two.

$$8,\underset{12\ 11\ 10}{6}\underset{9\ 8\ 7}{00},\underset{6\ 5\ 4}{000},\underset{3\ 2\ 1}{000}$$

23. B: An amphoteric substance can act as an acid or a base depending on the properties of the solute. Water is a common example and because of its amphoteric property, it serves as a universal solvent. Choice *A* is incorrect because it describes electrolytes. Choices *C* and *D* are incorrect because they both describe an acid.

24. C: To make a solution from a pure solid, the total molecular weight of the substance must be calculated and then the proper mass of the substance in grams must be added to water to make a solution. To calculate the total molecular weight, the individual molecular weights must be added. Finally, the mass of substance needed to make the solution can be calculated.

$$600mL\ CaCO_3 \times \frac{0.350\ m*l}{1000mL} \times \frac{100g\ CaCO_3}{1mol\ CaCO_3} = 21g\ CaCO_3$$

The calculations reveal that Choice *C* is the correct answer. All other reported values are incorrect.

25. C: Preparing a solution from a stock is simply a process of dilution by adding water to a certain amount of the stock. The amount of stock to use can be calculated using a formula and algebra:

$$V_S = \frac{M_D V_D}{M_S}$$

$$M_D = 1.8$$

$$V_D = 300ml$$

$$M_S = 15.0M$$

$$V_S = \frac{(1.80M)(300ml)}{15.0M} = 36.0\ ml$$

Because the given values are written to three significant figures, the answer should also be written in three significant figures, making Choice *C* the correct answer. The other answer choices are either incorrect values or reported to an incorrect number of significant figures.

Anatomy and Physiology

1. B: Proximal tubule → Loop of Henle → Collecting duct is correct. Kidneys filter blood using nephrons that span the outer renal cortex and inner renal medulla. The inner kidneys are composed of the renal pelvis, which collects urine and sends it to the bladder via the ureters. Filtrate first enters the filtering tube of the nephron via the glomerulus, a bundle of capillaries where blood fluid (but not cells) diffuses into the Bowman's capsule, the entryway into the kidney filtration canal. Bowman's capsule collects fluid, but the nephron actually starts filtering blood in the proximal tubule where necessary ions, nutrients, wastes, and (depending on blood osmolarity) water are absorbed or released. Also, blood pH is regulated, here, as the proximal tubule fine-tunes pH by utilizing the blood buffering system, adjusting amounts of hydrogen ions, bicarbonate, and ammonia in the filtrate. Down the loop of Henle in the renal medulla, the filtrate becomes more concentrated as water exits, while on the way back up the loop of Henle, ion concentration is regulated with ion channels. The distal tubule continues to regulate ion and water concentrations, and the collecting duct delivers the filtrate to the renal pelvis.

2. A: Motor neurons transmit signals from the CNS to effector tissues and organs, such as skeletal muscle and glands. Sensory neurons carry impulses from receptors in the extremities to the CNS. Interneurons relay impulses from neuron to neuron.

3. C: The cerebellum is important for balance and motor coordination. Aside from the brainstem and cerebellum, the outside portion of the brain is the cerebrum, which is the advanced operating system of the brain and is responsible for learning, emotion, memory, perception, and voluntary movement. The amygdala (emotions), language areas, and corpus collosum all exist within the cerebrum.

4. A: The exocrine portion of the pancreas (the majority of it) is an accessory organ to the digestive system (meaning that food never touches it—it is not part of the alimentary canal). It secretes bicarbonate to neutralize stomach acid and enzymes to aid in digestion. It also regulates blood sugar levels through the complementary action of insulin and glucagon that are located in the Islets of Langerhan (endocrine portion). *A* is incorrect because it is not the growth hormone that stimulates insulin secretion, but rather blood sugar levels.

5. D: The lymphatic system is composed of one-way vessels, lymph, and organs and is designed to filter pathogens and debris from the blood, return nutrients that have leaked from the blood, and maintain, and even stimulate, the immune system if necessary. It circulates lymph, a clear fluid filled with blood plasma that has leaked from capillary beds. The lymphatic system delivers lymph, a clear, colorless fluid, to the neck. It has several organs:

- Lymph nodes, which remove debris from lymph and forms lymphocytes
- The thymus, which develops lymphocytes
- The spleen, which removes pathogens from blood and makes lymphocytes
- Tonsils, which collect debris

The lymphatic system also absorbs lipids and fat-soluble vitamins from the gut and returns them to the circulatory system.

6. C: ADH secretion is correct. Antidiuretic hormone controls water reabsorption. In its presence, water is reabsorbed, and urine is more concentrated. When absent, water is excreted, and urine is dilute. It is a regulator of blood volume, not pH. The other choices do affect blood pH.

$$H_2O + CO_2 \leftrightarrow H_2CO_3 \leftrightarrow H^+ + HCO_3^-$$

This chemical reaction can be fine-tuned in order to tweak the pH. It's helpful to notice the hydrogen ion on the product side of the equation. The more hydrogen ions there are, the more acidic the blood is. Carbonic acid, the "middle-man," regulates blood by being a buffer. Exhaling releases carbon dioxide. This pushes the reaction to the left, which will decrease Hydrogen ions and make blood less acidic. Kidney regulation of bicarbonate will also shift the reaction to the left or right, raising or lowering pH as necessary.

Ammonia secreted by the proximal tubule of the nephron also regulates pH, since it will trap hydrogen ions and convert into ammonium ions. Reduced hydrogen ions make blood less acidic.

$$NH_3 + H^+ \leftrightarrow NH_4^+$$

7. D: The gland that regulates blood calcium levels is the parathyroid gland. Humans have four parathyroid glands located by the thyroid on each side of the neck, just below the larynx. Typical with the endocrine system, the parathyroid glands operate via feedback loops. If calcium in the blood is low, the parathyroid glands produce parathyroid hormone, which circulates to the bones and removes calcium. If calcium is high, they turn off parathyroid hormone production.

8. D: The hypothalamus is the link between the nervous and endocrine system. It receives information from the brain and sends signals to the pituitary gland, instructing it to release or inhibit release of hormones. Aside from its endocrine function, it controls body temperature, hunger, sleep, circadian rhythms, and is part of the limbic system.

9. C: When muscles contract, they pull bones together. They cannot push apart though, so they work in antagonistic pairs where they are on opposite sides of the bone.

When the bicep contracts, the arm bends and the tricep is relaxed; on the other hand, when the tricep contracts, the arm opens, and the bicep relaxes.

The quadriceps on the thigh straighten the knee; the hamstrings behind the thigh bend the knee.

The trapezius, rhomboid major, and rhomboid minor are muscles on the upper back that pull the shoulders back. The pectoralis major and minor (pecs) are on the chest and allow movement of the shoulder (throwing, lifting, rotating).

The gluteus maximus is the buttocks muscle and extends to the hip. It is the major of the glutes and is responsible for large movements like jumping. The gluteus medius and minimus stabilize the pelvis. The antagonist muscle to the gluteus maximus is the iliopasoas, the flexor muscles. Therefore, Choice C is incorrect since the glutes are not antagonistic muscles.

10. C: During muscle contractions, myosin cross-bridges attach via their globular heads to actin, then they swivel, and detach from actin filaments, causing the ends of the sarcomere to be pulled closer together. Choice A is incorrect, because it is essentially the opposite of this. Actin (the thin filament) does not attach to myosin (the thick filaments). Choice B is incorrect because the action potential is initiated when calcium leaves—rather than enters—the sarcoplasmic reticulum. Choice D is incorrect because fibers do not physically shorten. They slide past one another, shortening the distance between the origin and insertion of the muscle.

11. D: Cartilage and synovial fluid are the primary sources of cushioning to joints during impact. The proprioceptive system is responsible for body awareness, coordinated reflexes for balance, and modifying movements based on neural feedback.

12. A: Muscle spindles like in intrafusal muscle fibers, parallel to the direction of the extrafusal fibers. When a muscle is stretched, the embedded spindles are also stretched, activating sensory neurons in the spindles. This activation sends an impulse to the spinal cord, where the sensory neurons synapse with motor neurons. These motor neurons exit the spinal cord and travel back towards the limb, where they innervate with the extrafusal fibers, which receive the message to relax.

13. D: Passive range of motion assesses the non-contractile joint structures, such as ligaments, capsules, and fascia. Active range of motion would also assess the contractile elements (such as muscles and tendons) in addition to the non-contractile elements. Therefore, the specific muscles involved in knee flexion were not applicable to this question.

14. A: All three joint types given are synovial joints, allowing for a fair amount of movement (compared with fibrous and cartilaginous joints). Of the three given, hinge joints, such as the elbow, permit the least motion because they are uniaxial and permit movement in only one plane. Saddle joints and condyloid joints both have reciprocating surfaces that mate with one another and allow a variety of motions in numerous planes, but saddle joints, such as the thumb carpal metacarpal joint, allow more motion than condyloid joints. In saddle joints, two concave surfaces articulate, and in a condyloid joint, such as the wrist, a concave surface articulates with a convex surface, allowing motion in mainly two planes.

15. B: The smallest unit of a muscle fiber, sarcomeres, contain the actin and myosin proteins responsible for the mechanical process of muscle contractions. Located between two Z-lines, the actin and myosin filaments are configured in parallel, end-to-end, along the entire length of the myofibril. The sarcomere consists of four segments: the A-band, H-zone, I-band, and Z-line. The B-band and D-line are fictitious and are not components of a sarcomere.

16. D: Muscle fibers, also called muscle cells (i.e., myocytes), are long, striated, cylindrical cells that are approximately the diameter of a human hair (50 to 100 um), have many nuclei dispersed on the outside of the cell, and are covered by a fibrous membrane called the sarcolemma. Myofibrils, one of the smaller functional units within a myocyte, consist of long, thin (approximately 1/1000 mm) chains proteins. The smallest unit of a muscle fiber, a sarcomere, contains the actin and myosin proteins responsible for the mechanical process of muscle contractions.

17. A: The sarcoplasmic reticulum is a network of tubular channels and vesicles, which together provide structural integrity to the muscle fiber. The sarcoplasmic reticulum also acts as a calcium ion pump, moving Ca^{2+} ions from the sarcoplasm into the muscle fiber when the action potential reaches the cell. The Ca^{2+} binds with troponin, which causes the tropomyosin to move further into the double helix groove, allowing rapid binding of actin and myosin filaments and the power stroke that pulls the actin toward the center of the sarcomere, resulting in a contraction.

18. B: Choices I, II, and IV are correct. Here are the correct matches:

> Fibrous: sutures in skull
> Plane: intercarpal
> Saddle: thumb
> Hinge: elbow
> Condyloid: wrist
> Pivot: radial head on ulna
> Cartilaginous: pubic symphysis

19. C: Elbow extension and wrist flexion are movements that both take place in the sagittal plane (the sagittal plane cuts through the anterior and posterior of the body dividing the body into right and left regions). Shoulder abduction and neck left tilt movements both occur in the frontal plane.

20. B: Antagonists are muscles that oppose the action of the agonist (the primary muscle causing a motion). Hamstrings are the primary knee flexors (the agonists), and the quadriceps fire in opposition.

The gastrocnemius does cross the knee joint, so it is a knee flexor, although secondary to the hamstrings. Tibialis anterior is on the shin and is involved in dorsiflexion.

21. B: The respiratory system mediates the exchange of gas between the air and the circulating blood, mainly by the act of breathing. It filters, warms, and humidifies the air that gets breathed in and then passes it into the blood stream. The digestive system transforms food and liquids into energy and helps excrete waste from the body. Eliminating waste via the kidneys and bladder is a function of the urinary system.

22. A: The skeletal system consists of the 206 bones that make up the skeleton, as well as the cartilage, ligaments, and other connective tissues that stabilize the bones. The skeletal system provides structural support for the entire body, a framework for the soft tissues and organs to attach to, and acts as a protective barrier for some organs, such as the ribs protecting the heart and lungs, and the vertebrae protecting the spinal cord. The muscular system includes skeletal muscles, cardiac muscle, and the smooth muscles found on the inside of blood vessels. The endocrine system uses ductless glands to produce hormones that help maintain hemostasis, and the reproductive system is responsible for the production of egg and sperm cells.

23. A: It is most likely asthma. Any of the answer choices listed can cause heavy breathing. A blood clot in the lung (*B*) could cause this, but this would be very uncommon for a child. Choices *C* and *D* can both be ruled out because the question mentions that it occurs even when the patient is relaxing. Hyperventilation is usually caused by a panic attack or some sort of physical activity. Asthma often develops during childhood. It would stand to reason then that the child may have not yet been diagnosed. While asthma attacks can be caused by exercise they can also occur when a person is not exerting themselves.

24. A: The upper back has the one of the high densities of sweat glands of any area on the body. While palms, arms, and feet are often thought of as sweaty areas, they have relatively low amounts of sweat glands compared to other parts of the body. Remember that one of the purposes of sweat is thermoregulation, or controlling the temperature of the body. Regulating the temperature of one's core is more important than adjusting the temperature of one's extremities.

25. B: in a medical context, *genicular* or *geniculate* refer to something pertaining the knee. The term *geniculate* itself can be used in a more general context to refer to something bent sharply like the knee.

Physics

1. C: Electric charge can be transferred through touch of one physical object to another, induction by bringing a charged object near another object, and polarization, or the forcing of one charge to the end of an object in a centralized area.

2. A: Review the following conversion:

$$^0F = \frac{9}{5}(^0C) + 32$$

$$^0F = \frac{9}{5}(45) + 32$$

$$^0F = 113\ ^0F$$

Choices *B, C,* and *D* all incorporate a mistake in the order of operations necessary for this calculation: divide, multiply, and then add.

3. C: The force that opposes motion is called *friction*. It also provides the resistance necessary for walking, running, braking, etc. In order for something to slide down a ramp, it must be acted upon by a force stronger than that of friction. Choices *A* and *B* are not actual terms, and Choice *C* is the measure of mass multiplied by velocity ($p = mv$).

4. C: Using the equation for the conservation of momentum for an inelastic collision:

$$m_1 v_1 + m_2 v_2 = (m_1 + m_2)v_f$$

m_1 = 100 kg

m_2 = 110 kg

v_1 = 5 m/s

v_2 = 8 m/s

$$(100 \times 5) + (110 \times 8) = (100 + 110) \times v_f$$

$$(500) + (880) = (210) \times v_f$$

$$1380 = 210 \times v_f$$

$$1380/210 = v_f$$

$$v_f = 6.6 \text{ m/s}$$

Choices *A, B,* and *D* are answers created from possible mathematical errors when calculating the results.

5. D: The decibel scale is used to measure the intensity of sound waves. The decibel scale is a ratio of a particular sound's intensity to a standard value. Since it is a logarithmic scale, it is measured by a factor of 10. Choice *A* is the name of the effect experienced by an observer of a moving wave; Choice *B* is a particle in an atom; and Choice *C* is a unit for measuring power.

6. D: The weight of an object is equal to the mass of the object multiplied by gravity. According to Newton's Second Law of Motion, $F = m \times a$. Weight is the force resulting from a given situation, so the mass of the object needs to be multiplied by the acceleration of gravity on Earth: $W = m \times g$. Choice *A* is incorrect because, according to Newton's first law, all objects exert some force on each other, based on their distance from each other and their masses. This is seen in planets, which affect each other's paths and those of their moons. Choice *B* is incorrect because an object in motion or at rest can have inertia; inertia is the resistance of a physical object to change its state of motion. Choice *C* is incorrect because the mass of an object is a measurement of how much substance of there is to the object, while the weight is gravity's effect of the mass.

7. D: Polarization changes the oscillations of a wave and can alter the appearance in light waves. For example, polarized sunglasses remove the "glare" from sunlight by altering the oscillation pattern observed by the wearer. Choice *A*, reflection, is the bouncing back of a wave, such as in a mirror; Choice *B* is the bending of a wave as it travels from one medium to another, such as going from air to water; and Choice *C*, dispersion, is the spreading of a wave through a barrier or a prism.

8. A: An object moving in a circular motion also has momentum; it is called *angular momentum* and it is determined by the amount of rotational inertia, rotational velocity, and the distance of the mass from the axis of rotation. Objects exhibiting circular motion also demonstrate the conservation of angular momentum. This means that the angular momentum of a system is always constant, regardless of the placement of the mass. Rotational inertia can be affected by the distance of the mass of the object from the center of rotation (axis of rotation). The farther the mass is from the center of rotation, the slower the rotational velocity. While Choices *B*, *C*, and *D* are all conserved, none of them deal directly with circular motion, so they would not apply to the question.

9. D: Radiation can be transmitted through electromagnetic waves and needs no medium to travel; it can travel in a vacuum. This is how the Sun warms the Earth and it typically applies to large objects with great amounts of heat, or objects that have a large difference in their heat measurements. Choice *A*, convection, involves atoms or molecules traveling from areas of high concentration to those of low concentration and transferring energy or heat with them. Choice *B*, conduction, involves the touching or bumping of atoms or molecules to transfer energy or heat. Choice *C*, induction, deals with charges and does not apply to the transfer of energy or heat. Choices *A*, *B*, and *C* need a medium in which to travel, while radiation requires no medium.

10. C: Review the following:

$$a = \frac{\Delta v}{\Delta t}$$

$$a = \frac{15 - 0}{5 - 0}$$

$$a = \frac{15}{5}$$

$$= 3.0 \text{ m/s}^2$$

Choices *A* and *B* have the wrong units for acceleration; they are labeled with the units for velocity. Choices *B* and *D* integrate a miscalculation with the formula—multiplying, rather than dividing, 15 and 5.

HESI A2 Practice Test #3

Mathematics

1. Add 5,089 + 10,323
   a. 15,402
   b. 15,412
   c. 5,234
   d. 15,234

2. Add 103,678 + 487
   a. 103,191
   b. 103,550
   c. 104,265
   d. 104,165

3. Add 1.001 + 5.629
   a. 6.630
   b. 4.628
   c. 5.630
   d. 6.628

4. Add 143.77 + 5.2
   a. 138.57
   b. 148.97
   c. 138.97
   d. 148.57

5. Add and express in reduced form 5/12 + 4/9
   a. 9/17
   b. 1/3
   c. 31/36
   d. 3/5

6. Add and express in reduced form 14/33 + 10/11.
   a. 2/11
   b. 6/11
   c. 4/3
   d. 44/33

7. Subtract 9,576 – 891.
   a. 10,467
   b. 9,685
   c. 8,325
   d. 8,685

8. Subtract 112,076 – 1,243.
    a. 110,833
    b. 113,319
    c. 113,833
    d. 110,319

9. Subtract 50.888 – 13.091.
    a. 37.797
    b. 63.979
    c. 37.979
    d. 33,817

10. Subtract 701.1 – 52.33.
    a. 753.43
    b. 648.77
    c. 652.77
    d. 638.43

11. Subtract and express in reduced form 23/24 – 1/6.
    a. 22/18
    b. 11/9
    c. 19/24
    d. 4/5

12. Subtract and express in reduced form 43/45 – 11/15.
    a. 10/45
    b. 16/15
    c. 32/30
    d. 2/9

13. Multiply 578 × 15.
    a. 8,770
    b. 8,760
    c. 8,660
    d. 8,670

14. Multiply 13,114 × 191.
    a. 2,504,774
    b. 250,477
    c. 150,474
    d. 2,514,774

15. Multiply 12.4 × 0.2.
    a. 12.6
    b. 2.48
    c. 12.48
    d. 2.6

16. Multiply 1,987 × 0.05.
    a. 9.935
    b. 99.35
    c. 993.5
    d. 999.35

17. Multiply and reduce 15/23 × 54/127.
    a. 810/2,921
    b. 81/292
    c. 69/150
    d. 810/2929

18. Multiply and reduce 54/55 × 5/9.
    a. 59/64
    b. 270/495
    c. 6/11
    d. 5/9

19. Divide, express with a remainder 1,202 ÷ 44.
    a. 27 2/7
    b. 2 7/22
    c. 7 2/7
    d. 27 7/22

20. Divide, express with a remainder 188 ÷ 16.
    a. 1 3/4
    b . 111 3/4
    c. 10 3/4
    d. 11 3/4

21. Divide 702 ÷ 2.6.
    a. 27
    b. 207
    c. 2.7
    d. 270

22. Divide 1,015 ÷ 1.4.
    a. 7,250
    b. 725
    c. 7.25
    d. 72.50

23. Divide and reduce 26/55 ÷ 26/11.
    a. 52/11
    b. 26/11
    c. 1/5
    d. 2/5

24. Divide and reduce 4/13 ÷ 27/169.
   a. 52/27
   b. 51/27
   c. 52/29
   d. 51/29

25. What number is MCDXXXII?
   a. 142
   b. 1642
   c. 1632
   d. 1432

26. What number is CCLI?
   a. 1111
   b. 1151
   c. 151
   d. 251

27. Express 111 in Roman numerals.
   a. CCI
   b. CXI
   c. DDI
   d. DXI

28. Express 515 in Roman numerals.
   a. CVI
   b. DCV
   c. DXV
   d. VDV

29. Convert 1300 hours into a 12-hour clock time.
   a. 1:00 p.m.
   b. 11:00 a.m.
   c. 1:00 a.m.
   d. 11:00 p.m.

30. Convert 0830 hours into a 12-hour clock time.
   8:30 p.m.
   8:30 a.m.
   11:30 a.m.
   11:30 p.m.

31. What time is 5:00 p.m. in military (24-hour clock) time?
   a. 1500 hours
   b. 1700 hours
   c. 0500 hours
   d. 0700 hours

32. What time is 11:00am in military (24-hour clock) time?
    a. 0100 hours
    b. 1100 hours
    c. 1200 hours
    d. 0200 hours

33. The hospital has a nurse to patient ratio of 1:25. If there are a maximum of 325 patients admitted at a time, how many nurses are there?
    a. 13 nurses
    b. 25 nurses
    c. 325 nurses
    d. 12 nurses

34. A hospital has a bed to room ratio of 2: 1. If there are 145 rooms, how many beds are there?
    a. 145 beds
    b. 2 beds
    c. 90 beds
    d. 290 beds

35. Solve for X: $\frac{2x}{5} - 1 = 59$.
    a. 60
    b. 145
    c. 150
    d. 115

36. A National Hockey League store in the state of Michigan advertises 50% off all items. Sales tax in Michigan is 6%. How much would a hat originally priced at $32.99 and a jersey originally priced at $64.99 cost during this sale? Round to the nearest penny.
    a. $97.98
    b. $103.86
    c. $51.93
    d. $48.99

37. Store brand coffee beans cost $1.23 per pound. A local coffee bean roaster charges $1.98 per 1 ½ pounds. How much more would 5 pounds from the local roaster cost than 5 pounds of the store brand?
    a. $0.55
    b. $1.55
    c. $1.45
    d. $0.45

38. Paint Inc. charges $2000 for painting the first 1,800 feet of trim on a house and $1.00 per foot for each foot after. How much would it cost to paint a house with 3125 feet of trim?
    a. $3125
    b. $2000
    c. $5125
    d. $3325

39. A bucket can hold 11.4 liters of water. A kiddie pool needs 35 gallons of water to be full. How many times will the bucket need to be filled to fill the kiddie pool?

    a. 12

    b. 35

    c. 11

    d. 45

40. In Jim's school, there are 3 girls for every 2 boys. There are 650 students in total. Using this information, how many students are girls?

    a. 260

    b. 130

    c. 65

    d. 390

41. Convert 0.351 to a percentage.

    a. 3.51%

    b. 35.1%

    c. $\frac{351}{100}$

    d. 0.00351%

42. Convert $\frac{2}{9}$ to a percentage.

    a. 22%

    b. 4.5%

    c. 450%

    d. 0.22%

43. Convert 57% to a decimal.

    a. 570

    b. 5.70

    c. 0.06

    d. 0.57

44. What is 3 out of 8 expressed as a percent?

    a. 37.5%

    b. 37%

    c. 26.7%

    d. 2.67%

45. What is 39% of 164?

    a. 63.96%

    b. 23.78%

    c. 6,396%

    d. 2.38%

46. 32 is 25% of what number?
    a. 64
    b. 128
    c. 12.65
    d. 8

47. Convert $\frac{5}{8}$ to a decimal.
    a. 0.62
    b. 1.05
    c. 0.63
    d. 1.60

48. Change $3\frac{3}{5}$ to a decimal.
    a. 3.6
    b. 4.67
    c. 5.3
    d. 0.28

49. Change 0.56 to a fraction.
    a. 5.6/100
    b. 14/25
    c. 56/1000
    d. 56/10

50. Change 9.3 to a fraction.
    a. $9\frac{3}{7}$

    b. $\frac{903}{1000}$

    c. $\frac{9.03}{100}$

    d. $9\frac{3}{100}$

Reading Comprehension

Questions 1-6 are based on the following passage:

When researchers and engineers undertake a large-scale scientific project, they may end up making discoveries and developing technologies that have far wider uses than originally intended. This is especially true in NASA, one of the most influential and innovative scientific organizations in America. NASA *spinoff technology* refers to innovations originally developed for NASA space projects that are now used in a wide range of different commercial fields. Many consumers are unaware that products they are buying are based on NASA research! Spinoff technology proves that it is worthwhile to invest in science research because it could enrich people's lives in unexpected ways.

The first spinoff technology worth mentioning is baby food. In space, where astronauts have limited access to fresh food and fewer options about their daily meals, malnutrition is a serious concern. Consequently, NASA researchers were looking for ways to enhance the nutritional value of astronauts' food. Scientists found that a certain type of algae could be added to food, improving the food's neurological benefits. When experts in the commercial food industry learned of this algae's potential to boost brain health, they were quick to begin their own research. The nutritional substance from algae then developed into a product called life's DHA, which can be found in over 90% of infant food sold in America.

Another intriguing example of a spinoff technology can be found in fashion. People who are always dropping their sunglasses may have invested in a pair of sunglasses with scratch resistant lenses—that is, it's impossible to scratch the glass, even if the glasses are dropped on an abrasive surface. This innovation is incredibly advantageous for people who are clumsy, but most shoppers don't know that this technology was originally developed by NASA. Scientists first created scratch resistant glass to help protect costly and crucial equipment from getting scratched in space, especially the helmet visors in space suits. However, sunglasses companies later realized that this technology could be profitable for their products, and they licensed the technology from NASA.

1. What is the main purpose of this article?
    a. To advise consumers to do more research before making a purchase
    b. To persuade readers to support NASA research
    c. To tell a narrative about the history of space technology
    d. To define and describe instances of spinoff technology

2. What is the organizational structure of this article?
    a. A general definition followed by more specific examples
    b. A general opinion followed by supporting arguments
    c. An important moment in history followed by chronological details
    d. A popular misconception followed by counterevidence

3. Why did NASA scientists research algae?
    a. They already knew algae was healthy for babies.
    b. They were interested in how to grow food in space.
    c. They were looking for ways to add health benefits to food.
    d. They hoped to use it to protect expensive research equipment.

4. What does the word "neurological" mean in the second paragraph?
    a. Related to the body
    b. Related to the brain
    c. Related to vitamins
    d. Related to technology

5. Why does the author mention space suit helmets?
    a. To give an example of astronaut fashion
    b. To explain where sunglasses got their shape
    c. To explain how astronauts protect their eyes
    d. To give an example of valuable space equipment

6. Which statement would the author probably NOT agree with?
    a. Consumers don't always know the history of the products they are buying.
    b. Sometimes new innovations have unexpected applications.
    c. It is difficult to make money from scientific research.
    d. Space equipment is often very expensive.

Questions 7-14 are based on the following passage:

People who argue that William Shakespeare is not responsible for the plays attributed to his name are known as anti-Stratfordians (from the name of Shakespeare's birthplace, Stratford-upon-Avon). The most common anti-Stratfordian claim is that William Shakespeare simply was not educated enough or from a high enough social class to have written plays overflowing with references to such a wide range of subjects like history, the classics, religion, and international culture. William Shakespeare was the son of a glove-maker, he only had a basic grade school education, and he never set foot outside of England—so how could he have produced plays of such sophistication and imagination? How could he have written in such detail about historical figures and events, or about different cultures and locations around Europe? According to anti-Stratfordians, the depth of knowledge contained in Shakespeare's plays suggests a well-traveled writer from a wealthy background with a university education, not a countryside writer like Shakespeare. But in fact, there is not much substance to such speculation, and most anti-Stratfordian arguments can be refuted with a little background about Shakespeare's time and upbringing.

First of all, those who doubt Shakespeare's authorship often point to his common birth and brief education as stumbling blocks to his writerly genius. Although it is true that Shakespeare did not come from a noble class, his father was a very *successful* glove-maker and his mother was from a very wealthy land owning family—so while Shakespeare may have had a country upbringing, he was certainly from a well-off family and would have been educated accordingly. Also, even though he did not attend university, grade school education in Shakespeare's time was actually quite rigorous and exposed students to classic drama through writers like Seneca and Ovid. It is not unreasonable to believe that Shakespeare received a very solid foundation in poetry and literature from his early schooling.

Next, anti-Stratfordians tend to question how Shakespeare could write so extensively about countries and cultures he had never visited before (for instance, several of his most famous works like *Romeo and Juliet* and *The Merchant of Venice* were set in Italy, on the opposite side of Europe!). But again, this criticism does not hold up under scrutiny. For one thing, Shakespeare was living in London, a bustling metropolis of international trade, the most populous city in England, and a political and cultural hub of Europe. In the daily crowds of people, Shakespeare would certainly have been able to meet travelers from other countries and hear firsthand accounts of life in their home country. And, in addition to the influx of information from world travelers, this was also the age of the printing press, a jump in technology that made it possible to print and circulate books much more easily than in the past. This also allowed for a freer flow of information across different countries, allowing people to read about life and ideas from throughout Europe. One needn't travel the continent in order to learn and write about its culture.

7. What is the main purpose of this article?
    a. To explain two sides of an argument and allow readers to choose which side they agree with
    b. To encourage readers to be skeptical about the authorship of famous poems and plays
    c. To give historical background about an important literary figure
    d. To criticize a theory by presenting counterevidence

8. Which sentence contains the author's thesis?

    a. People who argue that William Shakespeare is not responsible for the plays attributed to his name are known as anti-Stratfordians.

    b. But in fact, there is not much substance to such speculation, and most anti-Stratfordian arguments can be refuted with a little background about Shakespeare's time and upbringing.

    c. It is not unreasonable to believe that Shakespeare received a very solid foundation in poetry and literature from his early schooling.

    d. Next, anti-Stratfordians tend to question how Shakespeare could write so extensively about countries and cultures he had never visited before.

9. In the first paragraph, "How could he have written in such detail about historical figures and events, or about different cultures and locations around Europe?" is an example of which of the following?

    a. Hyperbole

    b. Onomatopoeia

    c. Rhetorical question

    d. Appeal to authority

10. How does the author respond to the claim that Shakespeare was not well-educated because he did not attend university?

    a. By insisting upon Shakespeare's natural genius

    b. By explaining grade school curriculum in Shakespeare's time

    c. By comparing Shakespeare with other uneducated writers of his time

    d. By pointing out that Shakespeare's wealthy parents probably paid for private tutors

11. What does the word "bustling" in the third paragraph most nearly mean?

    a. Busy

    b. Foreign

    c. Expensive

    d. Undeveloped

12. What can be inferred from the article?

    a. Shakespeare's peers were jealous of his success and wanted to attack his reputation.

    b. Until recently, classic drama was only taught in universities.

    c. International travel was extremely rare in Shakespeare's time.

    d. In Shakespeare's time, glove-makers were not part of the upper class.

13. Why does the author mention *Romeo and Juliet*?

    a. It is Shakespeare's most famous play.

    b. It was inspired by Shakespeare's trip to Italy.

    c. It is an example of a play set outside of England.

    d. It was unpopular when Shakespeare first wrote it.

14. Which statement would the author probably agree with?

    a. It is possible to learn things from reading rather than from firsthand experience.

    b. If you want to be truly cultured, you need to travel the world

    c. People never become successful without a university education.

    d. All of the world's great art comes from Italy.

Questions 15-20 are based on the following passage:

This excerpt is adaptation from Abraham Lincoln's Address Delivered at the Dedication of the Cemetery at Gettysburg, November 19, 1863.

Four score and seven years ago our fathers brought forth on this continent, a new nation, conceived in liberty, and dedicated to the proposition that all men are created equal.

Now we are engaged in a great civil war, testing whether that nation, or any nation so conceived and so dedicated, can long endure. We are met on a great battlefield of that war. We have come to dedicate a portion of that field, as a final resting place for those who here gave their lives that this nation might live. It is altogether fitting and proper that we should do this.

But, in a larger sense, we cannot dedicate --- we cannot consecrate that we cannot hallow --- this ground. The brave men, living and dead, who struggled here, have consecrated it, far above our poor power to add or detract. The world will little note, nor long remember what we say here, but it can never forget what they did here. It is for us the living, rather, to be dedicated here to the unfinished work which they who fought here have thus far so nobly advanced. It is rather for us to be here and dedicated to the great task remaining before us--- that from these honored dead we take increased devotion to that cause for which they gave the last full measure of devotion --- that we here highly resolve that these dead shall not have died in vain --- that these this nation, under God, shall have a new birth of freedom--- and that government of people, by the people, for the people, shall not perish from the earth.

15. The best description for the phrase "Four score and seven years ago" is?
    a. A unit of measurement
    b. A period of time
    c. A literary movement
    d. A statement of political reform

16. What is the setting of this text?
    a. A battleship off of the coast of France
    b. A desert plain on the Sahara Desert
    c. A battlefield in a North American town
    d. The residence of Abraham Lincoln

17. Which war is Abraham Lincoln referring to in the following passage? "Now we are engaged in a great civil war, testing whether that nation, or any nation so conceived and so dedicated, can long endure."
    a. World War I
    b. The War of Spanish Succession
    c. World War II
    d. The American Civil War

18. What message is the author trying to convey through this address?
    a. The audience should consider the death of the people that fought in the war as an example and perpetuate the ideals of freedom that the soldiers died fighting for.
    b. The audience should honor the dead by establishing an annual memorial service.
    c. The audience should form a militia that would overturn the current political structure.
    d. The audience should forget the lives that were lost and discredit the soldiers.

19. Which rhetorical device is being used in the following passage?"...we here highly resolve that these dead shall not have died in vain --- that these this nation, under God, shall have a new birth of freedom--- and that government of people, by the people, for the people, shall not perish from the earth."

    a. Antimetabole

    b. Antiphrasis

    c. Anaphora

    d. Epiphora

20. What is the effect of Lincoln's statement in the following passage?: "But, in a larger sense, we cannot dedicate --- we cannot consecrate that we cannot hallow --- this ground. The brave men, living and dead, who struggled here, have consecrated it, far above our poor power to add or detract."

    a. His comparison emphasizes the great sacrifice of the soldiers who fought in the war.

    b. His comparison serves as a remainder of the inadequacies of his audience.

    c. His comparison serves as a catalyst for guilt and shame among audience members.

    d. His comparison attempts to illuminate the great differences between soldiers and civilians.

Questions 21-26 are based on the following passage.

This excerpt is an adaptation from The Immortal Cells of Henrietta Lacks by Rebecca Skloot.

Henrietta Lacks is an African American woman who died from an aggressive strain of cervical cancer. The word HeLa is used to refer to the cells grown from Henrietta Lacks's cervix. HeLa is known as the first immortal human cell line ever grown in culture.

The Cloning of HeLa

Today, when we hear the word clone, we imagine scientists creating entire living animals—like Dolly the famous cloned sheep—using DNA from one parent. But before the cloning of whole animals, there was the cloning of individual cells—Henrietta's cells.

To understand why cellular cloning was important, you need to know two things: First, HeLa didn't grow from one of Henrietta's cells. It grew from a sliver of her tumor, which was a cluster of cells. Second, cells often behave differently, even if they're all from the same sample, which means some grow faster than others, some produce more poliovirus, and some are resistant to certain antibiotics. Scientists wanted to grow cellular clones—lines of cells descended from individual cells—so they could harness those unique traits. With HeLa, a group of scientists in Colorado succeeded, and soon the world of science had not only HeLa but also its hundreds, then thousands, of clones.

The early cell culture and cloning technology developed using HeLa helped lead to many later advances that required the ability to grow single cells in culture, including isolating stem cells, cloning whole animals, and in vitro fertilization. Meanwhile, as the standard human cell in most labs, HeLa was also being used in research that would advance the new field of human genetics.

Researchers had long believed that human cells contained forty-eight chromosomes, the threads of DNA inside cells that contain all of our genetic information. But chromosomes clumped together, making it impossible to get an accurate count. Then, in 1953, a geneticist in Texas accidentally mixed the wrong liquid with HeLa and a few other cells, and it turned out to be a fortunate mistake. The chromosomes inside the cells swelled and spread out, and for the first time, scientists could see each of them clearly. That accidental discovery was the first of several developments that would allow two researchers from Spain and Sweden to discover that normal human cells have forty-six chromosomes.

Once scientists knew how many chromosomes people were supposed to have, they could tell when a person had too many or too few, which made it possible to diagnose genetic diseases. Researchers worldwide would soon begin identifying chromosomal disorders, discovering that patients with Down syndrome had an extra chromosome number 21, patients with Klinefelter syndrome had an extra sex chromosome, and those with Turner syndrome lacked all or part of one.

With all the new developments, demand for HeLa grew, and Tuskegee wasn't big enough to keep up. The owner of Microbiological Associates—a military man named Samuel Reader—knew nothing about science, but his business partner, Monroe Vincent, was a researcher who understood the potential market for cells. Many scientists needed cells, but few had the time or ability to grow them in large enough quantities. They just wanted to buy them. So together, Reader and Vincent used HeLa cells as the springboard to launch the first industrial-scale, for-profit cell distribution center.

21. The author's use of second person pronouns in the following text has all of the following effects except for? "To understand why cellular cloning was important, you need to know two things..."
   a. It personalizes the experience.
   b. It allows the reader to more easily understand the text.
   c. It encourages the reader to empathize with Henrietta Lack.
   d. It distances the reader from the text by overemphasizing the story.

22. The reference to "Dolly the famous cloned sheep" in the text points to which of the following facts?
   a. The HeLa cells research was not the only DNA-based research that has taken place.
   b. HeLa cells are the best evidence of cell mutation.
   c. HeLa cells provide no known evidence of the existence of immortal cells.
   d. Researchers doubt that HeLA cells exist.

23. What is the meaning of the word "harness" in the following text? "Scientists wanted to grow cellular clones—lines of cells descended from individual cells—so they could harness those unique traits."
   a. Tack
   b. Obtain
   c. Couple
   d. Duplicate

24. Where did HeLa cells initially originate?
   a. Within Henrietta Lack's heart
   b. Through Henrietta Lack's hair follicles
   c. Through DNA testing
   d. In a sliver of tumor from Henrietta Lack's cancerous cervical tissue

25. The discovery of HeLa cells has helped to further the scientific world through all of the following procedures except for?
   a. Isolating stem cells
   b. Cloning whole animals
   c. In vitro fertilization
   d. Separating Siamese twins

26. Normally developed humans have how many chromosomes?
    a. 48
    b. 47
    c. 46
    d. 41

Questions 27-32 are based on the following passage.

This excerpt is adaptation from The Ideas of Physics, Third Edition by Douglas C. Giancoli.

The Electric Battery

The events that led to the discovery of the battery are interesting; for not only was this an important discovery, but it also gave rise to a famous scientific debate between Alessandro Volta and Luigi Galvani, eventually involving many others in the scientific world.

In the 1780's, Galvani, a professor at the University of Bologna (thought to be the world's oldest university still in existence), carried out a long series of experiments on the contraction of a frog's leg muscle through electricity produced by a static-electricity machine. In the course of these investigations, Galvani found, much to his surprise, that contraction of the muscle could be produced by other means as well: when a brass hook was pressed into the frog's spinal cord and then hung from an iron railing that also touched the frog, the leg muscles again would contract. Upon further investigation, Galvani found that this strange but important phenomenon occurred for other pairs of metals as well.fr

Galvani believed that the source of the electric charge was in the frog muscle or nerve itself and the wire merely transmitted the charge to the proper points. When he published his work in 1791, he termed it "animal electricity." Many wondered, including Galvani himself, if he had discovered the long-sought "life-force."

Volta, at the University of Pavia 125 miles away, was at first skeptical of Galvani's results, but at the urging of his colleagues, he soon confirmed and extended those experiments. Volta doubted Galvani's idea of "animal electricity." Instead he came to believe that the source of the electricity was not in the animal, but rather in the contact between the two metals.

During Volta's careful research, he soon realized that a moist conductor, such as a frog muscle or moisture at the contact point of the two dissimilar metals, was necessary if the effect was to occur. He also saw that the contracting frog muscle was a sensitive instrument for detecting electric potential or voltage, in fact more sensitive than the best available electroscopes that he and others had developed. Volta's research showed that certain combinations of metals produced a greater effect than others.

Volta then conceived his greatest contribution to science. Between a disc of zinc and one of silver he placed a piece of cloth or paper soaked in salt solution or dilute acid and piled a "battery" of such couplings, one on top of another; this "pile" or "battery" produced a much increased potential difference. Indeed, when strips of metal connected to the two ends of the pile were brought close, a spark was produced. Volta had designed and built the first battery.

27. Which statement best details the central idea in this passage?
    a. It details the story of how the battery was originally developed.
    b. It delves into the mechanics of battery operated machines.
    c. It defines the far-reaching effects of battery usage throughout the world.
    d. It invites readers to create innovations that make the world more efficient.

28. Which definition most closely relates to the usage of the word "battery" in the passage?
    a. A group of objects that work in tandem to create an unified effect
    b. A log of assessments
    c. A series
    d. A violent encounter

29. Which type of text structure is employed in this following text?

During Volta's careful research, he soon realized that a moist conductor, such as a frog muscle or moisture at the contact point of the two dissimilar metals, was necessary if the effect was to occur. He also saw that the contracting frog muscle was a sensitive instrument for detecting electric potential or voltage, in fact more sensitive than the best available electroscopes that he and others had developed. Volta's research showed that certain combinations of metals produced a greater effect than others.

Between a disc of zinc and one of silver he placed a piece of cloth or paper soaked in salt solution or dilute acid and piled a "battery" of such couplings, one on top of another; this "pile" or "battery" produced a much increased potential difference. Indeed, when strips of metal connected to the two ends of the pile were brought close, a spark was produced. Volta had designed and built the first battery."

    a. Problem and solution
    b. Sequence
    c. Description
    d. Cause and effect

30. Which researcher was ultimately credited with creating "the first battery"?
    a. Galvani
    b. Pavia
    c. Volta
    d. Bologna

31. Which of the statements reflect information that one could reasonably infer based on Volta's scientific contributions concerning batteries?
    a. The researcher died in a state of shame and obscurity.
    b. Others researchers doubted his ability to create the first battery.
    c. The term "voltage" was created to recognize him for his contribution in the production of batteries.
    d. Researchers now use plastic to further technological advances in the field of electrical current conduction.

32. According to the following passage, which statement best describes the contrast between Volta and Galvani's theory concerning "animal electricity"? "Galvani believed that the source of the electric charge was in the frog muscle or nerve itself and the wire merely transmitted the charge to the proper points.

When he published his work in 1791, he termed it "animal electricity." Many wondered, including Galvani himself, if he had discovered the long-sought "life-force."

Volta, at the University of Pavia 125 miles away, was at first skeptical of Galvani's results, but at the urging of his colleagues, he soon confirmed and extended those experiments. Volta doubted Galvani's idea of "animal electricity." Instead he came to believe that the source of the electricity was not in the animal, but rather in the contact between the two metals."

    a. Galvani believed that only frogs were capable of serving as conductors for electricity.

    b. Volta doubted that animals possessed the intellect necessary to properly direct electricity to the proper source.

    c. Galvani believed that animals were carriers of the "life-force" necessary to conduct electricity while Volta felt that the meeting of metals was the catalyst for animal movement in the experiment.

    d. Both researchers held fast to the belief that their theories were the foremost and premiere research in the field.

Questions 33-37 are based upon the following passage.

This excerpt is adaptation from Mineralogy --- Encyclopedia International, Grolier

Mineralogy is the science of minerals, which are the naturally occurring elements and compounds that make up the solid parts of the universe. Mineralogy is usually considered in terms of materials in the Earth, but meteorites provide samples of minerals from outside the Earth.

A mineral may be defined as a naturally occurring, homogeneous solid, inorganically formed, with a definite chemical composition and an ordered atomic arrangement. The qualification *naturally occurring* is essential because it is possible to reproduce most minerals in the laboratory. For example, evaporating a solution of sodium chloride produces crystal indistinguishable from those of the mineral halite, but such laboratory-produced crystals are not minerals.

A *homogeneous solid* is one consisting of a single kind of material that cannot be separated into simpler compounds by any physical method. The requirement that a mineral be solid eliminates gases and liquids from consideration. Thus ice is a mineral (a very common one, especially at high altitudes and latitudes) but water is not. Some mineralogists dispute this restriction and would consider both water and native mercury (also a liquid) as minerals.

The restriction of minerals to *inorganically formed* substances eliminates those homogenous solids produced by animals and plants. Thus the shell of an oyster and the pearl inside, though both consist of calcium carbonate indistinguishable chemically or physically from the mineral aragonite comma are not usually considered minerals.

The requirement of a *definite chemical composition* implies that a mineral is a chemical compound, and the composition of a chemical compound is readily expressed by a formula. Mineral formulas may be simple or complex, depending upon the number of elements present and the proportions in which they are combined.

Minerals are crystalline solids, and the presence of an *ordered atomic arrangement* is the criterion of the crystalline state. Under favorable conditions of formation the ordered atomic arrangement is expressed in the external crystal form. In fact, the presence of an ordered atomic arrangement and crystalline solids was deduced from the external regularity of crystals by a French mineralogist, Abbé R. Haüy, early in the 19th century.

33. According to the text, an object or substance must have all of the following criteria to be considered a mineral except for?
   a. Be naturally occurring
   b. Be a homogeneous solid
   c. Be organically formed
   d. Have a definite chemical composition

34. One can deduce that French mineralogist Abbé R. Haüy specialized in what field of study?
   a. Geology
   b. Psychology
   c. Biology
   d. Botany

35. What is the definition of the word "homogeneous" as it appears in the following passage?

"A homogeneous solid is one consisting of a single kind of material that cannot be separated into simpler compounds by any physical method."
   a. Made of similar substances
   b. Differing in some areas
   c. Having a higher atomic mass
   d. Lacking necessary properties

36. The suffix -logy refers to?:
   a. The properties of
   b. The chemical makeup of
   c. The study of
   d. The classification of

37. The author included the counterargument in the following passage to achieve which following effect?

The requirement that a mineral be solid eliminates gases and liquids from consideration. Thus ice is a mineral (a very common one, especially at high altitudes and latitudes) but water is not. Some mineralogists dispute this restriction and would consider both water and native mercury (also a liquid) as minerals.
   a. To complicate the subject matter
   b. To express a bias
   c. To point to the fact that there are differing opinions in the field of mineralogy concerning the characteristics necessary to determine whether a substance or material is a mineral
   d. To create a new subsection of minerals

Questions 38-46 are based upon the following passage.

The Myth of Head Heat Loss

It has recently been brought to my attention that most people believe that 75% of your body heat is lost through your head. I had certainly heard this before, and am not going to attempt to say I didn't believe it when I first heard it. It is natural to be gullible to anything said with enough authority. But the "fact" that the majority of your body heat is lost through your head is a lie.

Let me explain. Heat loss is proportional to surface area exposed. An elephant loses a great deal more heat than an anteater, because it has a much greater surface area than an anteater. Each cell has mitochondria that produce energy in the form of heat, and it takes a lot more energy to run an elephant than an anteater.

So, each part of your body loses its proportional amount of heat in accordance with its surface area. The human torso probably loses the most heat, though the legs lose a significant amount as well. Some people have asked, "Why does it feel so much warmer when you cover your head than when you don't?" Well, that's because your head, because it is not clothed, is losing a lot of heat while the clothing on the rest of your body provides insulation. If you went outside with a hat and pants but no shirt, not only would you look stupid but your heat loss would be significantly greater because so much more of you would be exposed. So, if given the choice to cover your chest or your head in the cold, choose the chest. It could save your life.

38. The selection is told from what point of view?
    a. First
    b. Second
    c. Third
    d. Both A and B

39. What is the primary purpose of this passage?
    a. To provide evidence that disproves a myth
    b. To compare elephants and anteaters
    c. To explain why it is appropriate to wear clothes in winter
    d. To show how people are gullible

40. Which of the following best describes the main idea of the passage?
    a. It is better to wear a shirt than a hat
    b. Heat loss is proportional to surface area exposed
    c. It is natural to be gullible
    d. The human chest loses the most heat

41. Why does the author compare elephants and anteaters?
    a. To express an opinion
    b. To give an example that helps clarify the main point
    c. To show the differences between them
    d. To persuade why one is better than the other

42. The statement, "If you went outside with a hat and pants but no shirt, not only would you look stupid but your heat loss would be significantly greater because so much more of you would be exposed" is which of the following?
    a. An opinion
    b. A fact
    c. An opinion within a fact
    d. Neither

43. Which of the following best describes the tone of the passage?
    a. Harsh
    b. Angry
    c. Casual
    d. Indifferent

44. The author appeals to which branch of rhetoric to prove their case?
    a. Factual evidence
    b. Emotion
    c. Ethics and morals
    d. Author qualification

45. The selection is written in which of the following styles?
    a. Narrative
    b. Persuasive
    c. Informative
    d. Descriptive

46. Which of the following sentences provides the best evidence to support the main idea?
    a. "It is natural to be gullible to anything said with enough authority."
    b. "Each part of your body loses its proportional amount of heat in accordance with its surface area."
    c. "If given the choice to cover your chest or your head in the cold, choose the chest."
    d. "But the 'fact' that the majority of your body heat it lost through your head is a lie."

Vocabulary

1. What word meaning "on the opposite side" best fits in the following sentence? Although the patient's right knee had been hurting for a few months, he started experiencing _____ hip pain two weeks ago.
    a. Bilateral
    b. Ipsilateral
    c. Contralateral
    d. Alateral

2. Select the correct meaning of the underlined word in the following sentence. The patient's stomach appeared distended.
    a. Enlarged or expanded
    b. Sunken or concave
    c. Soft and flaccid
    d. Discolored or blotchy

3. What word meaning "rapidly or abruptly" best fits in the following sentence? When the school group arrived, the noise level in the waiting room rose _____.
    a. Concisely
    b. Precipitously
    c. Contingently
    d. Preemptively

4. What word meaning "open" best fits in the following sentence? After the obstruction was removed, the patient's bowel was _____.
    a. Patent
    b. Potent
    c. Evident
    d. Exude

5. What is the best definition of the word *amenorrhea*?
    a. Excessive bleeding
    b. Mental confusion
    c. Loss of appetite
    d. Absence of menstruation

6. Select the correct meaning of the underlined word in the following sentence. After the trauma, new symptoms of the woman's <u>latent</u> infection emerged.
    a. Chronic and debilitating
    b. Acute but not necessarily severe
    c. Present but not active or visible
    d. Uncontrollable or volatile

7. What word meaning "obvious" best fits in the following sentence? The patient's allergic reaction was _____, due to the widespread hives all over her extremities.
    a. Obsolete
    b. Covert
    c. Overt
    d. Colluded

8. Select the correct meaning of the underlined word in the following sentence. The nurse reported that the patient experienced <u>dyspnea</u> and dizziness.
    a. Difficulty breathing
    b. Difficulty sleeping
    c. Rapid pulse
    d. Nasal discharge

9. Select the correct meaning of the underlined word in the following sentence. The nurse explained the symptoms of the patient's <u>acute</u> illness and recommended increasing fluid intake.

    a. Serious with a poor prognosis
    b. Sudden or rapid onset
    c. Debilitating and contagious
    d. Chronic and slow to resolve

10. What word meaning "severe and harmful" best fits in the following sentence? The patient was quarantined because the doctor was concerned he had a _____ disease.
    a. Patent
    b. Innocuous
    c. Latent
    d. Virulent

11. What is the best definition of the word *adverse*?
    a. Unpredictable
    b. Agitated
    c. Undesirable
    d. Progressive

12. What word meaning "so gradual that it's hardly apparent" best fits in the following sentence? The nurse explained that atherosclerosis and coronary artery disease often have an _____ onset.
    a. Precipitous
    b. Insidious
    c. Incipient
    d. Paroxysmal

13. Select the correct meaning of the underlined word in the following sentence. The graduate student noted that the common symptoms of the condition were malaise, weight loss, and <u>anuria</u>.
    a. Lack of urine output
    b. Excessive urine production
    c. Memory loss
    d. Lack of usual reflexes

14. What word meaning "closer to the trunk" best fits in the following sentence? The knee is _____ to the ankle.
    a. Dorsal
    b. Distal
    c. Proximal
    d. Ventral

15. What word meaning "impenetrable" best fits in the following sentence? Due to the contagious nature of the patient's infection, the nursing staff was told to don _____ masks and gloves.
    a. Impotent
    b. Hygienic
    c. Impervious
    d. Impending

16. Select the correct meaning of the underlined word in the following sentence. The <u>etiology</u> of the disease is currently unknow.
    a. Prognosis or outlook
    b. Origin or cause
    c. Mechanism of transmission
    d. Incidence in the population

17. What word meaning "produced in the body" best fits in the following sentence? Endorphins are touted as acting as _____ opioids, to help reduce pain.
    a. Receptors
    b. Synthetic
    c. Exogenous
    d. Endogenous

18. What word meaning "feverish" best fits in the following sentence? The _____ baby was difficult to sooth.
   a. Febrile
   b. Futile
   c. Libel
   d. Liable

19. What is the best definition of the word *proliferated*?
   a. Multiplied or increased in number
   b. Responded to treatment
   c. Dwindled or decreased
   d. Expanded or grown in size

20. Select the correct meaning of the underlined word in the following sentence. The <u>viscosity</u> of the patient's synovial fluid was abnormal.
   a. A fluid's cellular and nutrient profile
   b. A fluid's thickness or resistance to flow
   c. A fluid's color and transparency
   d. A fluid's sedimentation rate

21. What word meaning "on one's back" best fits in the following sentence? The surgeon informed the patient that he would be _____ during the procedure.
   a. Prone
   b. Supine
   c. Dorsal
   d. Ventral

22. What is the best definition of the word *milieu*?
   a. Cytoplasm
   b. Organism
   c. Environment
   d. Autoclave

23. Select the correct meaning of the underlined word in the following sentence. The prognosis was undetermined because of the <u>aberrant</u> nature of his illness.
   a. Overt
   b. Grave
   c. Radical
   d. Abnormal

24. What word meaning "wound with irregular borders" best fits in the following sentence? The rock climber got a serious _____ on his arm when the boulder moved.
   a. Incision
   b. Laceration
   c. Contusion
   d. Avulsion

25. Select the correct meaning of the underlined word in the following sentence. The patient's father had a history of chronic <u>renal</u> disease.
   a. Relating to the pancreas

b. Relating to the liver

c. Relating to the kidney

d. Relating to hormones

26. Which word meaning "removal of necrotic tissue" best fits in the following sentence? The biker was hopeful that after his knee _____, he would be in less pain.

a. Debridement

b. Arthroscopy

c. Distension

d. Laparoscopy

27. Select the correct meaning of the underlined word in the following sentence. During her internship at the hospital, Cassandra got to triage a lot of patients.

a. Diagnose or identify a problem

b. Develop an effective treatment plan

c. Evaluate and gather relevant medical history

d. Sort based on problem severity

28. What word meaning "susceptible to" best fits in the following sentence? The malnourished child was _____ to rickets.

a. Impended

b. Invariable

c. Prognosticated

d. Predisposed

29. What word meaning "to widen or expand" best fits in the following sentence? The nitrous oxide was administered to _____ his blood vessels.

a. Dilute

b. Dilate

c. Occlude

d. Distill

30. Select the correct meaning of the underlined word in the following sentence. The nurse noted that the baby appeared indolent.

a. Underweight

b. Agitated

c. Lethargic

d. Alert

31. What word referring to "blood vessels that carry deoxygenated blood back to the heart" best fits in the following sentence? The nurse was concerned about possible occlusions in the patient's _____.

a. Capillaries

b. Arteries

c. Ventricles

d. Veins

32. Select the correct meaning of the underlined word in the following sentence. The medication had a buccal route of administration.
    a. Under the tongue
    b. In the rectum
    c. Through the nasal cavity
    d. Inside the cheek

33. What is the best definition of the word *instructor*?
    a. Pupil
    b. Teacher
    c. Survivor
    d. Dictator

34. What is the best definition of the word *expectorate*?
    a. To cough out phlegm
    b. To suppress a phlegm production
    c. To stifle a cough
    d. Yellowish or green sputum

35. What is the best definition of the word *residence*?
    a. Home
    b. Area
    c. Plan
    d. Resist

36. What is the best definition of the word *relinquish*?
    a. Stop repeatedly
    b. Give again
    c. Punish again
    d. Cease claim

37. What is the best definition of the word *germinate*?
    a. Lengthen
    b. Infect
    c. Develop
    d. Ail

38. What is the best definition of the word *indemnity?*
    a. Insurance
    b. Punishment
    c. Affinity
    d. Insolation

39. Select the correct meaning of the underlined word in the following sentence. Immediately after the holiday, staff interest grew rampant.
    a. Stagnant
    b. Mildly
    c. Unrestrained
    d. Wearily

40. Select the correct meaning of the underlined word in the following sentence. An increased pupil size is considered an <u>ominous</u> sign.
  - a. Unequivocal
  - b. Promising
  - c. Auspicious
  - d. Threatening

41. What word meaning "low blood sugar" best fits in the following sentence? A patient with diabetes did not receive breakfast so the nurse was concerned he might have _____.
  - a. Hypoglycemia
  - b. Ketoacidosis
  - c. Diabetic coma
  - d. Hyperglycemia

42. What is the best definition of the word *observed*?
  - a. Watched
  - b. Hunted
  - c. Scared
  - d. Sold

43. What word meaning "sleepy yet arousable to verbal stimuli" best fits in the following sentence? The _____ patient was difficult to move to into the room.
  - a. Comatose
  - b. Delirious
  - c. Somnolent
  - d. Stuporous

44. What word meaning "coughing up blood" best fits in the following sentence? A patient with tuberculosis should be monitored for _____.
  - a. Hematopoiesis
  - b. Hemoptysis
  - c. Hematemesis
  - d. Hematochezia

45. What is the best definition of the word *engorge*?
  - a. Nourish
  - b. Squeeze
  - c. Consume
  - d. Swell

46. What word meaning "mourning after loss" best fits in the following sentence. The nurse referred the mother to _____ counseling.
  - a. Bereavement
  - b. Disposition
  - c. Depression
  - d. Belligerent

47. What word meaning "excessive thirst" best fits in the following sentence? A common side effect of antispasmodics is _____.
    a. Anurea
    b. Polyploidy
    c. Polydipsia
    d. Polyurea

48. What is the best definition of the word *sentient*?
    a. Kind and genial
    b. Aging or dying
    c. Able to feel or perceive
    d. Nostalgic

49. Select the correct meaning of the underlined word in the following sentence. The patient had a history of anxiety, emphysema, and a <u>peptic</u> ulcer.
    a. Relating to ingestion
    b. Relating to defecation
    c. Relating to digestion
    d. Relating to the pancreas

50. What word meaning "a muscle contraction that does not cause a change in muscle length" best fits in the following sentence? The strength training protocol called for many _____ exercises.
    a. Isometric
    b. Isotonic
    c. Isokinetic
    d. Plyometric

Grammar

For questions 1–18, select the answer choice that best replaces the underlined portion of the sentence. If the original sentence is best, select Choice A, NO CHANGE.

1. <u>Some of universities provide internship or apprentice opportunities</u> for the students enrolled in aircraft engineer programs.
    a. NO CHANGE
    b. Some of universities provided internship or apprentice opportunities
    c. Some of universities provide internship or apprenticeship opportunities
    d. Some universities provide internship or apprenticeship opportunities

2. These advanced offices oftentimes require a Professional Engineering (PE) license which can be obtained through additional college courses, professional experience, and acceptable scores on the Fundamentals of Engineering (FE) and Professional Engineering (PE) standardized assessments.

    a. NO CHANGE

    b. These advanced positions oftentimes require acceptable scores on the Fundamentals of Engineering (FE) and Professional Engineering (PE) standardized assessments in order to achieve a Professional Engineering (PE) license. Additional college courses and professional experience help.

    c. These advanced offices oftentimes require acceptable scores on the Fundamentals of Engineering (FE) and Professional Engineering (PE) standardized assessments to gain the Professional Engineering (PE) license which can be obtained through additional college courses, professional experience.

    d. These advanced positions oftentimes require a Professional Engineering (PE) license which is obtained by acceptable scores on the Fundamentals of Engineering (FE) and Professional Engineering (PE) standardized assessments. Further education and professional experience can help prepare for the assessments.

3. This level of expertise <u>allows</u> aircraft engineers to apply mathematical equations and scientific processes to aeronautical and aerospace issues or inventions.

    a. NO CHANGE

    b. Inhibits

    c. Requires

    d. Should

4. <u>For example, aircraft engineers may test, design, and construct flying vessels such as airplanes, space shuttles, and missile weapons.</u>

    a. NO CHANGE

    b. Therefore,

    c. However,

    d. Furthermore,

5. <u>In May 2015, the United States Bureau of Labor Statistics (BLS) reported that the median annual salary of aircraft engineers was $107, 830.</u>

    a. NO CHANGE

    b. May of 2015, the United States Bureau of Labor Statistics (BLS) reported that the median annual salary of aircraft engineers was $107, 830.

    c. In May of 2015 the United States Bureau of Labor Statistics (BLS) reported that the median annual salary of aircraft engineers was $107, 830.

    d. In May, 2015, the United States Bureau of Labor Statistics (BLS) reported that the median annual salary of aircraft engineers was $107, 830.

6. <u>Conversely,</u> employment opportunities for aircraft engineers are projected to decrease by 2 percent by 2024.

    a. NO CHANGE

    b. Similarly,

    c. In other words,

    d. Accordingly,

7. <u>Employment opportunities for aircraft engineers are projected to decrease by 2 percent by 2024.</u>
    a. NO CHANGE
    b. Employment opportunities for aircraft engineers will be projected to decrease by 2 percent in 2024.
    c. Employment opportunities for aircraft engineers is projected to decrease by 2 percent in 2024.
    d. Employment opportunities for aircraft engineers were projected to decrease by 2 percent in 2024.

8. <u>Bin Laden orchestrated the attacks as a response to what he felt was American injustice against Islam and hatred towards Muslims.</u>
    a. NO CHANGE
    b. Bin Laden orchestrated the attacks as a response to what he felt was American injustice against Islam, and hatred towards Muslims.
    c. Bin Laden orchestrated the attacks, as a response to what he felt was American injustice against Islam and hatred towards Muslims.
    d. Bin Laden orchestrated the attacks as responding to what he felt was American injustice against Islam and hatred towards Muslims.

9. Which of the following would NOT be an appropriate replacement for the underlined portion of the following sentence? The <u>crash was initially thought to be</u> a freak accident.
    a. First crash was thought to be
    b. Initial crash was thought to be
    c. Thought was that the initial crash
    d. Initial thought was that the crash was

10. Although the passengers were successful in <u>diverging</u> the plane, it crashed in a western Pennsylvania field and killed everyone on board.
    a. NO CHANGE
    b. Diverting
    c. Converging
    d. Distracting

11. <u>Although often associated with devastation, not all flooding results</u> in adverse circumstances.
    a. NO CHANGE
    b. Although often associated with devastation not all flooding results
    c. Although often associated with devastation. Not all flooding results
    d. While often associated with devastation, not all flooding results

12. The Taliban, a group of fundamental Muslims who protected Osama bin Laden, was overthrown on December 9, 2001. However, the war continued in order to defeat insurgency campaigns in neighboring countries.

    a. NO CHANGE

    b. The Taliban was overthrown on December 9, 2001. They were a group of fundamental Muslims who protected Osama bin Laden. However, the war continued in order to defeat insurgency campaigns in neighboring countries.

    c. The Taliban, a group of fundamental Muslims who protected Osama bin Laden, on December 9, 2001 was overthrown. However, the war continued in order to defeat insurgency campaigns in neighboring countries.

    d. Osama bin Laden's fundamental Muslims who protected him were called the Taliban and overthrown on December 9, 2001. Yet the war continued in order to defeat the insurgency campaigns in neighboring countries.

13. Fred Hampton desired to see lasting social change for African American people through nonviolent means and community recognition. As a result, he became an African American activist during the American Civil Rights Movement and led the Chicago chapter of the Black Panther Party.

    a. NO CHANGE

    b. As a result he became an African American activist

    c. As a result: he became an African American activist

    d. As a result of, he became an African American activist

14. Hampton soon became the leader of the Chicago chapter of the BPP where he organized rallies, taught political education classes, and established a free medical clinic.

    a. NO CHANGE

    b. As the leader of the BPP, Hampton: organized rallies, taught political education classes, and established a free medical clinic.

    c. As the leader of the BPP, Hampton; organized rallies, taught political education classes, and established a free medical clinic.

    d. As the leader of the BPP, Hampton—organized rallies, taught political education classes, and established a medical free clinic.

15. Such technologies can also be used to project the severity of an anticipated flood.

    a. NO CHANGE

    b. Projecting

    c. Project

    d. Projected

16. How could this sentence be rewritten without losing its original meaning? O'Neal provided the FBI with detailed floor plans of the BPP's headquarters, identifying the exact location of Hampton's bed.

    a. NO CHANGE

    b. O'Neal provided the FBI with detailed floor plans of the BPP's headquarters, which identified the exact location of Hampton's bed.

    c. O'Neal provided the FBI with detailed floor plans and Hampton's bed.

    d. O'Neal identified the exact location of Hampton's bed that provided the FBI with detailed floor plans of the BPP's headquarters.

17. Which of the following revisions can be made to the following sentence that will still maintain the original meaning while making the sentence more concise? <u>Flooding can occur slowly or within seconds and can submerge small regions or extend over vast areas of land.</u>
    a. NO CHANGE
    b. Flooding can either be slow or occur within seconds. It doesn't take long to submerge small regions or extend vast areas of land.
    c. Flooding occurs slowly or rapidly submerging vast areas of land.
    d. Vast areas of land can be flooded slowly or within seconds.

18. They fear that the melting of icebergs will cause the <u>oceans levels</u> to rise and flood coastal regions.
    a. NO CHANGE
    b. Ocean levels
    c. Ocean's levels
    d. Levels of the oceans

19. Which of these examples shows incorrect use of subject-verb agreement?
    a. Neither of the cars are parked on the street.
    b. Both of my kids are going to camp this summer.
    c. Any of your friends are welcome to join us on the trip in November.
    d. Each of the clothing options is appropriate for the job interview.

20. When it gets warm in the spring, _____ and _____ like to go fishing at Cobbs Creek. Which of the following word pairs should be used in the blanks above?
    a. me, him
    b. he, I
    c. him, I
    d. he, me

21. The realtor showed _____ and _____ a house on Wednesday afternoon. Which of the following pronoun pairs should be used in the blanks above?
    a. She, I
    b. She, me
    c. Me, her
    d. Her, me

22. A teacher notices that, when students are talking to each other between classes, they are using their own unique vocabulary words and expressions to talk about their daily lives. When the teacher hears these non-standard words that are specific to one age or cultural group, what type of language is she listening to?
    a. Slang
    b. Jargon
    c. Dialect
    d. Vernacular

23. A teacher wants to counsel a student about using the word *ain't* in a research paper for a high school English class. What advice should the teacher give?

    a. *Ain't* is not in the dictionary, so it isn't a word.

    b. Because the student isn't in college yet, *ain't* is an appropriate expression for a high school writer.

    c. *Ain't* is incorrect English and should not be part of a serious student's vocabulary because it sounds uneducated.

    d. *Ain't* is a colloquial expression, and while it may be appropriate in a conversational setting, it is not standard in academic writing.

24. What is the structure of the following sentence?

    The restaurant is unconventional because it serves both Chicago style pizza and New York style pizza.

    a. Simple
    b. Compound
    c. Complex
    d. Compound-complex

25. The following sentence contains what kind of error?

    This summer, I'm planning to travel to Italy, take a Mediterranean cruise, going to Pompeii, and eat a lot of Italian food.

    a. Parallelism
    b. Sentence fragment
    c. Misplaced modifier
    d. Subject-verb agreement

26. The following sentence contains what kind of error?

    Forgetting that he was supposed to meet his girlfriend for dinner, Anita was mad when Fred showed up late.

    a. Parallelism
    b. Run-on sentence
    c. Misplaced modifier
    d. Subject-verb agreement

27. The following sentence contains what kind of error?

    Some workers use all their sick leave, other workers cash out their leave.

    a. Parallelism
    b. Comma splice
    c. Sentence fragment
    d. Subject-verb agreement

28. A student writes the following in an essay:

Protestors filled the streets of the city. Because they were dissatisfied with the government's leadership.

Which of the following is an appropriately-punctuated correction for this sentence?

a. Protestors filled the streets of the city, because they were dissatisfied with the government's leadership.

b. Protesters, filled the streets of the city, because they were dissatisfied with the government's leadership.

c. Because they were dissatisfied with the government's leadership protestors filled the streets of the city.

d. Protestors filled the streets of the city because they were dissatisfied with the government's leadership.

29. What is the part of speech of the underlined word in the sentence?

We need to come up with a fresh <u>approach</u> to this problem.

a. Noun
b. Verb
c. Adverb
d. Adjective

30. What is the part of speech of the underlined word in the sentence?

Investigators conducted an <u>exhaustive</u> inquiry into the accusations of corruption.

a. Noun
b. Verb
c. Adverb
d. Adjective

31. The underlined portion of the sentence is an example of which sentence component?

New students should report <u>to the student center</u>.

a. Dependent clause
b. Adverbial phrase
c. Adjective clause
d. Noun phrase

32. Which word choices will correctly complete the sentence?

Increasing the price of bus fares has had a greater [affect / effect] on ridership [then / than] expected.

a. affect; then
b. affect; than
c. effect; then
d. effect; than

33. The following is an example of what type of sentence?

Although I wished it were summer, I accepted the change of seasons, and I started to appreciate the fall.

a. Compound
b. Simple
c. Complex
d. Compound-Complex

34. A student reads the following sentence:

A hundred years ago, automobiles were rare, but now cars are ubiquitous.

However, she doesn't know what the word *ubiquitous* means. Which key context clue is essential to decipher the word's meaning?

a. Ago
b. Cars
c. Now
d. Rare

35. Which word in the following sentence is a proper noun?

People think the Statue of Liberty is an awesome sight.

a. People
b. Statue of Liberty
c. Awesome
d. Sight

36. Which word in the following sentence is a plural noun?

The black kitten was the girl's choice from the litter of kittens.

a. Kitten
b. Girl's
c. Choice
d. Kittens

37. Which pronoun makes the following sentence grammatically correct?

_____ ordered the flowers?

a. Whose
b. Whom
c. Who
d. Who've

38. Which pronoun makes the following sentence grammatically correct?

The giraffe nudged _____ baby.

a. it's
b. hers
c. their
d. its

39. What is the word *several* in the following sentence called?

     Several are laughing loudly on the bus.
   a. Singular indefinite pronoun
   b. Plural indefinite pronoun
   c. Singular objective pronoun
   d. Indefinite adjective

40. Which word in the following sentence is an adjective?

     The connoisseur slowly enjoyed the delectable meal.
   a. Delectable
   b. Connoisseur
   c. Slowly
   d. Enjoyed

41. Which choice identifies all of the prepositions in the following sentence?

     We went down by the water, near the lake, before dawn, to see the pretty sunrise.
   a. Went, to see, pretty
   b. By, near, before
   c. Water, lake, dawn, sunrise
   d. We, down, the, pretty

42. Which sentence has an interjection?
   a. The cookie was full of chocolaty goodness.
   b. Well, Carrie didn't like the cookie.
   c. Can't you see that cookie is broken?
   d. That's too bad, but I'll still eat it!

43. Identify the complete subject in the following sentence.

     The heaviest green bike is mine.
   a. bike
   b. green bike
   c. heaviest green bike
   d. is mine

44. Identify the complete predicate in the following sentence.

     My house is the yellow one at the end of the street.
   a. My house
   b. is the yellow one
   c. at the end of the street.
   d. is the yellow one at the end of the street.

45. Which sentence shows incorrect subject/verb agreement?
   a. All of the kittens in the litter show their courage.
   b. The black kitten pounce on the ball of yarn.
   c. The calico kitten eats voraciously.
   d. My favorite kitten snuggles with its mother.

46. What is the indirect object in the following sentence?
     Calysta brought her mother the beautiful stained-glass lamp.
    a. Stained-glass lamp
    b. Brought
    c. Her mother
    d. Beautiful

47. Which sentence is grammatically correct?
    a. They're on their way to New Jersey but there not there yet.
    b. Their on their way to New Jersey but they're not there yet.
    c. They're on their way to New Jersey but they're not there yet.
    d. They're on their way to New Jersey but there not their yet.

48. Identify the prepositional phrase in the following sentence.
     For the longest time, I have wanted to learn to roller skate.
    a. I have wanted
    b. wanted to learn
    c. learn to roller skate
    d. For the longest time

49. Identify the sentence structure of the following sentence.
     The weight of the world was on his shoulders, so he took a long walk.
    a. Simple sentence
    b. Compound sentence
    c. Complex sentence
    d. Compound-complex sentence

50. Identify the sentence structure of the following sentence.
     The last thing she wanted to do was see the Eiffel Tower before the flight.
    a. Simple sentence
    b. Compound sentence
    c. Complex sentence
    d. Compound-complex sentence

Biology

1. What is the theory that certain physical and behavioral survival traits give a species an evolutionary advantage called?
    a. Gradualism
    b. Evolutionary Advantage
    c. Punctuated Equilibrium
    d. Natural Selection

2. Which of the following is NOT a unique property of water?
    a. High cohesion and adhesion
    b. High surface tension
    c. High density upon melting
    d. High freezing point

3. What is a metabolic reaction that releases energy called?
    a. Catabolic
    b. Carbolic
    c. Anabolic
    d. Endothermic

4. What organic compounds facilitate chemical reactions by lowering activation energy?
    a. Carbohydrates
    b. Lipids
    c. Enzymes
    d. Nucleotides

5. Which structure is exclusively in eukaryotic cells?
    a. Cell wall
    b. Nucleus
    c. Cell membrane
    d. Vacuole

6. Which of these is NOT found in the cell nucleus?
    a. Golgi complex
    b. Chromosomes
    c. Nucleolus
    d. Chromatin

7. Which is the cellular organelle used for digestion to recycle materials?
    a. Golgi apparatus
    b. Lysosome
    c. Centriole
    d. Mitochondria

8. What are the energy-generating structures of the cell called?
    a. Nucleoplasms
    b. Mitochondria
    c. Golgi Apparatus
    d. Ribosomes

9. Which is a component of plant cells not found in animal cells?
    a. Nucleus
    b. Plastid
    c. Cell membrane
    d. Cytoplasm

10. Diffusion and osmosis are examples of what type of transport mechanism?
    a. Active
    b. Passive
    c. Extracellular
    d. Intracellular

11. The combination of alleles of an organism, when expressed, manifests as the organism's _____.
    a. genotype.
    b. phenotype.
    c. gender.
    d. karyotype.

12. Which of the choices below are the reproductive cells produced by meiosis?
    a. Genes
    b. Alleles
    c. Chromatids
    d. Gametes

13. What is the process of cell division in somatic (most body) cells called?
    a. Mitosis
    b. Meiosis
    c. Respiration
    d. Cytogenesis

14. Which is true regarding DNA?
    a. It is the genetic code.
    b. It provides energy.
    c. It is single-stranded.
    d. All of the above.

15. What does NOT happen at stomata?
    a. Carbon dioxide enters.
    b. Water exits due to transpiration.
    c. Oxygen exits.
    d. Glucose exits.

16. What is an alteration in the normal gene sequence called?
    a. DNA mutation
    b. Gene migration
    c. Polygenetic inheritance
    d. Incomplete dominance

17. Blood type is a trait determined by multiple alleles, and two of them are co-dominant: I^A codes for A blood and I^B codes for B blood. i codes for O blood and is recessive to both. If an A heterozygote individual and an O individual have a child, what is the probably that the child will have A blood?
    a. 25%
    b. 50%
    c. 75%
    d. 100%

18. What are the building blocks of DNA referred to as?
    a. Helices
    b. Proteins
    c. Genes
    d. Nucleotides

19. Which statement is NOT true about RNA?
    a. It can be single-stranded.
    b. It has ribose sugar.
    c. It has uracil.
    d. It only exists in three forms.

20. Water has many unique properties due to its unique structure. Which of the following do not play a role in water's unique properties?
    a. Hydrogen bonding between molecules
    b. Polarity within one molecule
    c. Molecules held apart in solid state
    d. Equal sharing of electrons

21. What is the term used for the set of metabolic reactions that convert chemical bonds to energy in the form of ATP?
    a. Photosynthesis
    b. Reproduction
    c. Active transport
    d. Cellular respiration

22. What step happens first in protein synthesis?
    a. mRNA is pulled into the ribosome.
    b. Exons are spliced out of mRNA in processing.
    c. tRNA delivers amino acids.
    d. mRNA makes a complementary DNA copy.

23. What is the idea that evolution involves long periods of stasis and short periods of rapid change?
    a. Natural selection
    b. Punctuated equilibrium
    c. Gradualism
    d. Commensalism

24. Which function below is NOT one of lipids?
    a. Provides cellular instructions
    b. Can be chemical messages
    c. Provides energy
    d. Composes cell membranes

25. What is the cell structure responsible for protein synthesis called?
    a. DNA
    b. Golgi Apparatus
    c. Nucleus
    d. Ribosome

Chemistry

1. Which number below is equal to 1.0×10^{-2}?
    a. 1
    b. 10
    c. 100
    d. .01

2. Which is the metric prefix for 10^{-3}?
    a. Milli
    b. Centi
    c. Micro
    d. Deci

3. What is the temperature in Fahrenheit when it is 35°C outside?
    a. 67°F
    b. 95°F
    c. 63°F
    d. 75°F

4. How are a sodium atom and a sodium isotope different?
    a. The isotope has a different number of protons.
    b. The isotope has a different number of neutrons.
    c. The isotope has a different number of electrons.
    d. The isotope has a different atomic number.

5. Which statement is true about nonmetals?
    a. They form cations.
    b. They form covalent bonds.
    c. They are mostly absent from organic compounds.
    d. They are all diatomic.

6. What is the basic unit of matter?
    a. Elementary particle
    b. Atom
    c. Molecule
    d. Photon

7. Which particle is responsible for all chemical reactions?
    a. Electrons
    b. Neutrons
    c. Protons
    d. Orbitals

8. Which of these give atoms a negative charge?
    a. Electrons
    b. Neutrons
    c. Protons
    d. Orbital

9. How are similar chemical properties of elements grouped on the periodic table?
    a. In rows according to their total configuration of electrons
    b. In columns according to the electron configuration in their outer shells
    c. In rows according to the electron configuration in their outer shells
    d. In columns according to their total configurations of electrons

10. In a chemical equation, the reactants are on which side of the arrow?
    a. Right
    b. Left
    c. Neither right nor left
    d. Both right and left

11. What does the law of conservation of mass state?
    a. All matter is equally created.
    b. Matter changes but is not created.
    c. Matter can be changed, and new matter can be created
    d. Matter can be created, but not changed.

12. Which factors decrease solubility of solids?
    a. Heating
    b. Agitation
    c. Large Surface area
    d. Decreasing solvent

13. What information is used to calculate the quantity of solute in a solution?
    a. Molarity of the solution
    b. Equivalence point
    c. Limiting reactant
    d. Theoretical yield

14. How does adding salt to water affect its boiling point?
    a. It increases it.
    b. It has no effect.
    c. It decreases it.
    d. It prevents it from boiling.

15. What is the effect of pressure on a liquid solution?
    a. It decreases solubility.
    b. It increases solubility.
    c. It has little effect on solubility.
    d. It has the same effect as with a gaseous solution.

16. Nonpolar molecules must have what kind regions?
    a. Hydrophilic
    b. Hydrophobic
    c. Hydrolytic
    d. Hydrochloric

17. Which of these is a substance that increases the rate of a chemical reaction?
    a. Catalyst
    b. Brine
    c. Solvent
    d. Inhibitor

18. Which of the following are composed of chains of amino acids?
    a. Lipids
    b. Nucleic Acids
    c. Proteins
    d. Carbohydrates

19. What is the balance of the following combustion equation?

$$\_C_2 H_{10} + \_O_2 \rightarrow \_H_2O + \_CO_2$$

    a. 1:5:5:2
    b. 1:9:5:2
    c. 2: 9:10:4
    d. 2:5:10:4

20. Which type of bonding results from transferring electrons between atoms?
    a. Ionic bonding
    b. Covalent bonding
    c. Hydrogen bonding
    d. Dipole interactions

21. Which substance is oxidized in the following reaction?

$$4Fe + 3O_2 \rightarrow 2Fe_2O_3$$

    a. Fe
    b. O
    c. O_2
    d. Fe_2O_3

22. Which statements are true regarding nuclear fission?
    I. Splitting of heavy nuclei
    II. Utilized in power plants
    III. Occurs on the sun
    a. I only
    b. II and III only
    c. I and II only
    d. III only

23. Which type of nuclear decay is occurring in the equation below?

$$U_{92}^{236} \rightarrow He_2^4 + Th_{90}^{232}$$

    a. Alpha
    b. Beta
    c. Gamma
    d. Delta

24. Which statement is true about the pH of a solution?
    a. A solution cannot have a pH less than 1.
    b. The more hydroxide ions there are in the solution, the higher the pH will be.
    c. If an acid has a pH of greater than -2, it is considered a weak acid.
    d. A solution with a pH of 2 has ten times the amount of hydronium ions than a solution with a pH of 1.

25. Which radioactive particle is the most penetrating and damaging and is used to treat cancer in radiation?
    a. Alpha
    b. Beta
    c. Gamma
    d. Delta

Anatomy and Physiology

1. Which statement about white blood cells is true?
    a. B cells are responsible for antibody production.
    b. White blood cells are made in the white/yellow cartilage before they enter the bloodstream.
    c. Platelets, a special class of white blood cell, function to clot blood and stop bleeding.
    d. The majority of white blood cells only activate during the age of puberty, which explains why children and the elderly are particularly susceptible to disease.

2. Which locations in the digestive system are sites of chemical digestion?
    I. Mouth
    II. Stomach
    III. Small Intestine

    a. II only
    b. III only
    c. II and III only
    d. I, II, and III

3. Which of the following are functions of the urinary system?
  I. Synthesizing calcitriol and secreting erythropoietin
  II. Regulating the concentrations of sodium, potassium, chloride, calcium, and other ions
  III. Reabsorbing or secreting hydrogen ions and bicarbonate
  IV. Detecting reductions in blood volume and pressure

  a. I, II, and III
  b. II and III
  c. II, III, and IV
  d. All of the above

4. If the pressure in the pulmonary artery is increased above normal, which chamber of the heart will be affected first?
  a. The right atrium
  b. The left atrium
  c. The right ventricle
  d. The left ventricle

5. What is the purpose of sodium bicarbonate when released into the lumen of the small intestine?
  a. It works to chemically digest fats in the chyme.
  b. It decreases the pH of the chyme so as to prevent harm to the intestine.
  c. It works to chemically digest proteins in the chyme.
  d. It increases the pH of the chyme so as to prevent harm to the intestine.

6. Which of the following describes a reflex arc?
  a. The storage and recall of memory
  b. The maintenance of visual and auditory acuity
  c. The autoregulation of heart rate and blood pressure
  d. A stimulus and response controlled by the spinal cord

7. Ligaments connect what?
  a. Muscle to muscle
  b. Bone to bone
  c. Bone to muscle
  d. Muscle to tendon

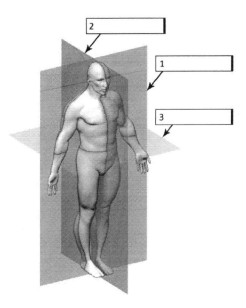

8. Identify the correct sequence of the 3 primary body planes as numbered 1, 2, and 3 in the above image.

    a. Plane 1 is coronal, plane 2 is sagittal, and plane 3 is transverse.

    b. Plane 1 is sagittal, plane 2 is coronal, and plane 3 is medial.

    c. Plane 1 is coronal, plane 2 is sagittal, and plane 3 is medial.

    d. Plane 1 is sagittal, plane 2 is coronal, and plane 3 is transverse.

9. Which of the following is NOT a major function of the respiratory system in humans?

    a. It provides a large surface area for gas exchange of oxygen and carbon dioxide.

    b. It helps regulate the blood's pH.

    c. It helps cushion the heart against jarring motions.

    d. It is responsible for vocalization.

10. Which of the following is NOT a function of the forebrain?

    a. To regulate blood pressure and heart rate

    b. To perceive and interpret emotional responses like fear and anger

    c. To perceive and interpret visual input from the eyes

    d. To integrate voluntary movement

11. A patient's body is not properly filtering blood. Which of the following body parts is most likely malfunctioning?

    a. Medulla

    B. Heart

    C. Nephrons

    D. Renal cortex

12. A pediatrician notes that an infant's cartilage is disappearing and being replaced by bone. What process has the doctor observed?
   a. Mineralization
   b. Ossification
   c. Osteoporosis
   d. Calcification

13. Which of the following creates sperm?
   a. Prostate gland
   b. Seminal vesicles
   c. Scrotum
   d. Seminiferous tubules

14. Which of the following functions corresponds to the parasympathetic nervous system?
   a. It stimulates the fight-or-flight response.
   b. It increases heart rate.
   c. It stimulates digestion.
   d. It increases bronchiole dilation.

15. Which of the following is the gland that helps regulate calcium levels?
   a. Osteotoid gland
   b. Pineal gland
   c. Parathyroid glands
   d. Thymus gland

16. Which of the following is the best unit to measure the amount of blood in the human body?
   a. Ounces
   b. Liters
   c. Milliliters
   d. Pounds

17. What type of vessel carries oxygen-rich blood from the heart to other tissues of the body?
   a. Veins
   b. Intestines
   c. Bronchioles
   d. Arteries

18. The somatic nervous system is responsible for which of the following?
   a. Breathing
   b. Thought
   c. Movement
   d. Fear

19. Which blood component is chiefly responsible for clotting?
   a. Platelets
   b. Red blood cells
   c. Antigens
   d. Plasma cells

20. What is the function of the sinuses?
    a. To trap the many airborne pathogens
    b. To direct air down the trachea rather than the esophagus
    c. To warm, humidify, and filter air
    d. To sweep away pathogens and direct them toward the top of the trachea

21. Which of the following structures acts like a funnel by delivering the urine from the millions of the collecting tubules to the ureters?
    a. The renal pelvis
    b. The renal cortex
    c. The renal medulla
    d. Bowman's capsule

22. A cluster of capillaries that functions as the main filter of the blood entering the kidney is known as which of the following?
    a. The Bowman's capsule
    b. The Loop of Henle
    c. The glomerulus
    d. The nephron

23. What is the name for the sac-shaped structures in which carbon dioxide and oxygen exchange takes place?
    a. Kidneys
    b. Medulla oblongata
    c. Alveoli
    d. Bronchioles

24. The muscular tube that connects the outer surface to the cervix in a woman's birth canal is referred to as which of the following?
    a. The uterus
    b. The cervix
    c. The vagina
    d. The ovaries

25. Which of the following organs functions both as an endocrine and exocrine gland?
    a. The kidney
    b. The spleen
    c. The pancreas
    d. The stomach

Physics

1. Velocity is a measure of which of the following?
    a. Speed with direction
    b. The change in speed over the change in time
    c. Acceleration with direction
    d. All of the above

2. What is the definition of acceleration?
   a. The rate at which an object moves
   b. The rate of change in velocity
   c. Speed in a given direction
   d. The velocity of an object multiplied by its mass

3. Which of the following is NOT one of Newton's three laws of motion?
   a. An object at rest tends to stay at rest, and an object in motion tends to stay in motion
   b. $E = mc^2$
   c. For every action, there is an equal and opposite reaction
   d. $F = ma$

4. For circular motion, what is the name of the actual force pulling toward the axis of rotation?
   a. Centrifugal force
   b. Gravity
   c. Centripetal force
   d. No force is acting

5. The energy of motion is also referred to as what?
   a. Potential energy
   b. Kinetic energy
   c. Electric energy
   d. Electromagnetic energy

6. What is the purpose of a wave?
   a. To carry matter
   b. To transfer energy
   c. To do work
   d. To slow down matter

7. What is the term for when a wave bends?
   a. Refraction
   b. Diffraction
   c. Reflection
   d. Convection

8. Which of the following reside in the nucleus of an atom?
   a. Protons and neutrons
   b. Neutrons and electrons
   c. Electrons and ions
   d. Ions and protons

9. How does electrical energy flow?
   a. From objects with lesser potential energy to objects with greater potential energy
   b. Equally between objects with equal potential energy
   c. From objects with greater potential energy to objects with lesser potential energy
   d. From objects with greater magnetic energy to objects with greater electrical energy

10. Which of the following is true regarding electromagnetism?
    a. Opposite charges attract
    b. Like charges attract
    c. Opposite charge are neutral towards one another
    d. Like charges are neutral towards one another

Answer Explanations

Mathematics

1. B: 15,412

Set up the problem and add each column, starting on the far right (ones). Add, carrying anything over 9 into the next column to the left. Solve from right to left.

2. D: 104,165

Set up the problem and add each column, starting on the far right (ones). Add, carrying anything over 9 into the next column to the left. Solve from right to left.

3. A: 6.630

Set up the problem, with the larger number on top and numbers lined up at the decimal. Add, carrying anything over 9 into the next column to the left. Solve from right to left.

4. B: 148.97

Set up the problem, with the larger number on top and numbers lined up at the decimal. Insert 0 in any blank spots to the right of the decimal as placeholders. Add, carrying anything over 9 into the next column to the left.

5. C: 31/36

Set up the problem and find a common denominator for both fractions.

$$\frac{5}{12} + \frac{4}{9}$$

Multiply each fraction across by 1 to convert to a common denominator.

$$\frac{5}{12} \times \frac{3}{3} + \frac{4}{9} \times \frac{4}{4}$$

Once over the same denominator, add across the top. The total is over the common denominator.

$$\frac{15 + 16}{36} = \frac{31}{36}$$

6. C: 4/3

Set up the problem and find a common denominator for both fractions.

$$\frac{14}{33} + \frac{10}{11}$$

Multiply each fraction across by 1 to convert to a common denominator

$$\frac{14}{33} \times \frac{1}{1} + \frac{10}{11} \times \frac{3}{3}$$

Once over the same denominator, add across the top. The total is over the common denominator.

$$\frac{14 + 30}{33} = \frac{44}{33}$$

Reduce by dividing both numerator and denominator by 11.

$$\frac{44 \div 11}{33 \div 11} = \frac{4}{3}$$

7. D: 8,685

Set up the problem, with the larger number on top. Begin subtracting with the far right column (ones). Borrow 10 from the column to the left, when necessary.

8. A: 110,833

Set up the problem, with the larger number on top. Begin subtracting with the far right column (ones). Borrow 10 from the column to the left, when necessary.

9. A: 37.797

Set up the problem, larger number on top and numbers lined up at the decimal. Begin subtracting with the far right column. Borrow 10 from the column to the left, when necessary.

10. B: 648.77

Set up the problem, with the larger number on top and numbers lined up at the decimal. Insert 0 in any blank spots to the right of the decimal as placeholders. Begin subtracting with the far right column. Borrow 10 from the column to the left, when necessary.

11. C: 19/24

Set up the problem and find a common denominator for both fractions.

$$\frac{23}{24} - \frac{1}{6}$$

Multiply each fraction across by 1 to convert to a common denominator.

$$\frac{23}{24} \times \frac{1}{1} - \frac{1}{6} \times \frac{4}{4}$$

Once over the same denominator, subtract across the top.

$$\frac{23 - 4}{24} = \frac{19}{24}$$

12. D: 2/9

Set up the problem and find a common denominator for both fractions.

$$\frac{43}{45} - \frac{11}{15}$$

Multiply each fraction across by 1 to convert to a common denominator.

$$\frac{43}{45} \times \frac{1}{1} - \frac{11}{15} \times \frac{3}{3}$$

Once over the same denominator, subtract across the top.

$$\frac{43 - 33}{45} = \frac{10}{45}$$

Reduce.

$$\frac{10 \div 5}{45 \div 5} = \frac{2}{9}$$

13. D: 8670

Line up the numbers (the number with the most digits on top) to multiply. Begin with the left column on top and the left column on bottom (8 × 5).

Move one column left on top and multiply by the far right column on the bottom. Remember to add the carry over after you multiply.

Starting on the far right column, on top, repeat this pattern for the next number left on the bottom. Write the answers below the first line of answers. Remember to begin with a zero placeholder.

Continue the pattern.

Add the answer rows together, making sure they are still lined up correctly.

14. A: 2,504,774

Line up the numbers (the number with the most digits on top) to multiply. Begin with the right column on top and the right column on bottom.

Move one column left on top and multiply by the far right column on the bottom. Remember to add the carry over after you multiply. Continue that pattern for each of the numbers on the top row.

Starting on the far right column on top repeat this pattern for the next number left on the bottom. Write the answers below the first line of answers; remember to begin with a zero placeholder. Continue for each number in the top row.

Starting on the far right column on top, repeat this pattern for the next number left on the bottom. Write the answers below the first line of answers. Remember to begin with zero placeholders.

Once completed, ensure the answer rows are lined up correctly, then add.

15. B: 2.48

Set up the problem, with the larger number on top. Multiply as if there are no decimal places. Add the answer rows together. Count the number of decimal places that were in the original numbers ($1 + 1 = 2$).

Place the decimal 2 places the right for the final solution.

16. B: 99.35

Set up the problem, with the larger number on top. Multiply as if there are no decimal places. Add the answer rows together. Count the number of decimal places that were in the original numbers (2).

Place the decimal in that many spots from the right for the final solution.

17. A: $810/2921$

Line up the fractions.

$$\frac{15}{23} \times \frac{54}{127}$$

Multiply across the top and across the bottom.

$$\frac{15 \times 54}{23 \times 127} = \frac{810}{2921}$$

18. C: $6/11$

Line up the fractions.

$$\frac{54}{55} \times \frac{5}{9}$$

Reduce fractions through cross-canceling.

$$\frac{6}{11} \times \frac{1}{1}$$

Multiply across the top and across the bottom.

$$\frac{6 \times 1}{11 \times 1} = \frac{6}{11}$$

19. D: 27 7/22

Set up the division problem.

$$44\overline{)1202}$$

44 does not go into 1 or 12 but will go into 120 so start there.

$$
\begin{array}{r}
27 \\
44\overline{)1202} \\
-88 \\
\hline
322 \\
-308 \\
\hline
14
\end{array}
$$

The answer is 27 14/44.

Reduce the fraction for the final answer.

27 7/22

20. D: 11 3/4

Set up the division problem.

$$16\overline{)188}$$

16 does not go into 1 but does go into 18 so start there.

$$
\begin{array}{r}
11 \\
16\overline{)188} \\
-16 \\
\hline
28 \\
-16 \\
\hline
12
\end{array}
$$

The result is 11 12/16

Reduce the fraction for the final answer.

11 3/4

21. D: 270

Set up the division problem.

$$2.6\overline{)702}$$

Move the decimal over one place to the right in both numbers.

$$26\overline{)7020}$$

26 does not go into 7 but does go into 70 so start there.

$$
\begin{array}{r}
270 \\
26\overline{)7020} \\
-52 \\
\hline
182 \\
-182 \\
\hline
0
\end{array}
$$

The result is 270

22. B: 725

Set up the division problem.

$$1.4\overline{)1015}$$

Move the decimal over one place to the right in both numbers.

$$14\overline{)10150}$$

14 does not go into 1 or 10 but does go into 101 so start there.

$$
\begin{array}{r}
725 \\
14\overline{)10150} \\
-98 \\
\hline
35 \\
-28 \\
\hline
70 \\
-70 \\
\hline
0
\end{array}
$$

The result is 725.

23. C: 1/5

Set up the division problem.

$$\frac{26}{55} \div \frac{26}{11}$$

Flip the second fraction and multiply.

$$\frac{26}{55} \times \frac{11}{26}$$

Simplify and reduce with cross multiplication.

$$\frac{1}{5} \times \frac{1}{1}$$

Multiply across the top and across the bottom.

$$\frac{1 \times 1}{5 \times 1} = \frac{1}{5}$$

24. A: 52/27

Set up the division problem.

$$\frac{4}{13} \div \frac{27}{169}$$

Flip the second fraction and multiply.

$$\frac{4}{13} \times \frac{169}{27}$$

Simplify and reduce with cross multiplication.

$$\frac{4}{1} \times \frac{13}{27}$$

Multiply across the top and across the bottom to solve.

$$\frac{4 \times 13}{1 \times 27} = \frac{52}{27}$$

25. D: 1432

Break down the roman numerals into parts.

MCDXXXII

M is equal to 1000.

C is before D and is smaller than D, so it means D - C.

CD = 500 - 100 = 400

Add the following:

XXX = 10 + 10 + 10 = 30

II = 1 + 1 = 2

Add all parts.

1000 + 400 + 30 + 2 = 1432

26. D: 251

Break down the roman numerals into parts.

CCLI

Add the following.

CC = 100 + 100 = 200

L = 50

I = 1

Add all parts.

200 + 50 + 1 = 251

27. B: CXI

Break down the number into parts.

111 = 100 + 10 + 1

100 is represented by C or 100 = C

10 is represented by X or 10 = X

1 is represented by 1 or 1 = I

Combine the Roman numerals.

CXI

28. C: DXV

Break down the number into parts.

515 = 500 + 10 + 5

500 is represented by D or 500 = D

10 is represented by X or 10 = X

5 is represented by V or 5 = V

Combine the Roman numerals.

DXV

29. A: 1:00 p.m.

Since military time starts with 0100 at 1:00 a.m., add 12 to get to 1300 hours, or 1:00 p.m.

30. B: 8:30 a.m.

Anything before 1200 would be in the a.m. hours of a 12-hour clock, so 0830 hours is 8:30 a.m.

31. B: 1700 hours

To convert 5:00 p.m. into 24-hour time, add 12 to 5.

32. B: 1100 hours

Anything before noon converts over from its a.m. value.

33. A: 13 nurses

Using the given information of 1 nurse to 25 patients and 325 patients, set up an equation to solve for number of nurses (N):

$$\frac{N}{325} = \frac{1}{25}$$

Multiply both sides by 325 to get N by itself on one side.

$$\frac{N}{1} = \frac{325}{25} = 13 \; nurses$$

34. D: 290 beds

Using the given information of 2 beds to 1 room and 145 rooms, set up an equation to solve for number of beds (B):

$$\frac{B}{145} = \frac{2}{1}$$

Multiply both sides by 145 to get B by itself on one side.

$$\frac{B}{1} = \frac{290}{1} = 290 \; beds$$

35. C: X = 150

Set up the initial equation.

$$\frac{2X}{5} - 1 = 59$$

Add 1 to both sides.

$$\frac{2X}{5} - 1 + 1 = 59 + 1$$

Multiply both sides by 5/2.

$$\frac{2X}{5} \times \frac{5}{2} = 60 \times \frac{5}{2} = 150$$

$$X = 150$$

36. C: $51.93

List the givens.

$$Tax = 6.0\% = 0.06$$

$$Sale = 50\% = 0.5$$

$$Hat = \$32.99$$

$$Jersey = \$64.99$$

Calculate the sales prices.

$$Hat\ Sale = 0.5\,(32.99) = 16.495$$

$$Jersey\ Sale = 0.5\,(64.99) = 32.495$$

Total the sales prices.

$$Hat\ sale + jersey\ sale = 16.495 + 32.495 = 48.99$$

Calculate the tax and add it to the total sales prices.

$$Total\ after\ tax = 48.99 + (48.99\ x\ 0.06) = \$51.93$$

37. D: $0.45

List the givens.

$$Store\ coffee = \$1.23/lbs$$

$$Local\ roaster\ coffee = \$1.98/1.5\ lbs$$

Calculate the cost for 5 lbs of store brand.

$$\frac{\$1.23}{1\ lbs} \times 5\ lbs = \$6.15$$

Calculate the cost for 5 lbs of the local roaster.

$$\frac{\$1.98}{1.5\ lbs} \times 5\ lbs = \$6.60$$

Subtract to find the difference in price for 5 lbs.

$$\begin{array}{r} \$6.60 \\ -\ \underline{\$6.15} \\ \$0.45 \end{array}$$

38. D: $3,325

List the givens.

$$1,800 \ ft. = \$2,000$$

$$Cost \ after \ 1,800 \ ft. = \$1.00/ft.$$

Find how many feet left after the first 1,800 ft.

$$
\begin{array}{r}
3,125 \text{ ft.} \\
- \quad 1,800 \text{ ft.} \\
\hline
1,325 \text{ ft.}
\end{array}
$$

Calculate the cost for the feet over 1,800 ft.

$$1,325 \ ft. \times \frac{\$1.00}{1 \ ft} = \$1,325$$

Total for entire cost.

$$\$2,000 + \$1,325 = \$3,325$$

39. A: 12

Calculate how many gallons the bucket holds.

$$11.4 \ L \ \times \ \frac{1 \ gal}{3.8 \ L} = 3 \ gal$$

Now how many buckets to fill the pool which needs 35 gallons.

$$35/3 = 11.67$$

Since the amount is more than 11 but less than 12, we must fill the bucket 12 times.

40. D: Three girls for every two boys can be expressed as a ratio: 3:2. This can be visualized as splitting the school into 5 groups: 3 girl groups and 2 boy groups. The number of students which are in each group can be found by dividing the total number of students by 5:

650 divided by 5 equals 1 part, or 130 students per group

To find the total number of girls, multiply the number of students per group (130) by how the number of girl groups in the school (3). This equals 390, answer *D*.

41. B: 35.1%

To convert from a decimal to a percentage, the decimal needs to be moved two places to right. In this case, that makes 0.351 become 35.1%.

42. B: 22%

Converting from a fraction to a percentage generally involves two steps. First, the fraction needs to be converted to a decimal.

Divide 2 by 9 which results in $0.\overline{22}$. The top line indicates that the decimal actually goes on forever with an endless amount of 2's.

Second, the decimal needs to be moved two places to the right:

$$22\%$$

43. D: 0.57

To convert from a percentage to a decimal, or vice versa, you always need to move the decimal two places. A percentage like 57% has an invisible decimal after the 7, like this:

$$57.\%$$

That decimal then needs to be moved two places to the left to get:

$$0.57$$

44. A: 37.5%

Solve this by setting up the percent formula:

$$\frac{3}{8} = \frac{\%}{100}$$

Multiply 3 by 100 to get 300 . Then divide 300 by 8:

$$300 \div 8 = 37.5\%$$

Note that with the percent formula, 37.5 is automatically a percentage and does not need to have any further conversions.

45. A: 63.96%

This question involves the percent formula. Since, we're beginning with a percent, also known as a number over 100, we'll put 39 on the right side of the equation:

$$\frac{x}{164} = \frac{39}{100}$$

Now, multiple 164 and 39 to get 6,396, which then needs to be divided by 100.

$$6,396 \div 100 = 63.96$$

46. B: 128

This question involves the percent formula.

$$\frac{32}{x} = \frac{25}{100}$$

We multiply the diagonal numbers, 32 and 100, to get 3,200. Dividing by the remaining number, 25, gives us 128.

The percent formula does not have to be used for a question like this. Since 25% is ¼ of 100, you know that 32 needs to be multiplied by 4, which yields 128.

47. C: 0.63

Divide 5 by 8, which results in 0.63.

48. A: 3.6

Divide 3 by 5 to get 0.6 and add that to the whole number 3, to get 3.6. An alternative is to incorporate the whole number 3 earlier on by creating an improper fraction: 18/5. Then dividing 18 by 5 to get 3.6.

49. B: 14/25

Since 0.56 goes to the hundredths place, it can be placed over 100:

$$\frac{56}{100}$$

Essentially, the way we got there is by multiplying the numerator and denominator by 100:

$$\frac{0.56}{1} \times \frac{100}{100} = \frac{56}{100}$$

Then, the fraction can be simplified down to 14/25:

$$\frac{56}{100} \div \frac{4}{4} = \frac{14}{25}$$

50. D: $9\frac{3}{10}$

To convert a decimal to a fraction, remember that any number to the left of the decimal point will be a whole number. Then, sense 0.3 goes to the tenths place, it can be placed over 10.

Reading Comprehension

1. D: To define and describe instances of spinoff technology. This is an example of a purpose question— *why* did the author write this? The article contains facts, definitions, and other objective information without telling a story or arguing an opinion. In this case, the purpose of the article is to inform the reader. The only answer choice that is related to giving information is answer Choice *D*: to define and describe.

2. A: A general definition followed by more specific examples. This organization question asks readers to analyze the structure of the essay. The topic of the essay is about spinoff technology; the first paragraph gives a general definition of the concept, while the following two paragraphs offer more detailed examples to help illustrate this idea.

3. C: They were looking for ways to add health benefits to food. This reading comprehension question can be answered based on the second paragraph—scientists were concerned about astronauts' nutrition and began researching useful nutritional supplements. A in particular is not true because it reverses the order of discovery (first NASA identified algae for astronaut use, and then it was further developed for use in baby food).

4. B: Related to the brain. This vocabulary question could be answered based on the reader's prior knowledge; but even for readers who have never encountered the word "neurological" before, the passage does provide context clues. The very next sentence talks about "this algae's potential to boost brain health," which is a paraphrase of "neurological benefits." From this context, readers should be able to infer that "neurological" is related to the brain.

5. D: To give an example of valuable space equipment. This purpose question requires readers to understand the relevance of the given detail. In this case, the author mentions "costly and crucial equipment" before mentioning space suit visors, which are given as an example of something that is very valuable. A is not correct because fashion is only related to sunglasses, not to NASA equipment. B can be eliminated because it is simply not mentioned in the passage. While C seems like it could be a true statement, it is also not relevant to what is being explained by the author.

6. C: It is difficult to make money from scientific research. The article gives several examples of how businesses have been able to capitalize on NASA research, so it is unlikely that the author would agree with this statement. Evidence for the other answer choices can be found in the article: A, the author mentions that "many consumers are unaware that products they are buying are based on NASA research"; B is a general definition of spinoff technology; and D is mentioned in the final paragraph.

7. D: To criticize a theory by presenting counterevidence. The author mentions anti-Stratfordian arguments in the first paragraph, but then goes on to debunk these theories with more facts about Shakespeare's life in the second and third paragraphs. A is not correct because, while the author does present arguments from both sides, the author is far from unbiased; in fact, the author clearly disagrees with anti-Stratfordians. B is also not correct because it is more closely aligned to the beliefs of anti-Stratfordians, whom the author disagrees with. C can be eliminated because, while it is true that the author gives historical background, the main purpose of the article is using that information to disprove a theory.

8. B: But in fact, there is not much substance to such speculation, and most anti-Stratfordian arguments can be refuted with a little background about Shakespeare's time and upbringing. The thesis is a statement that contains the author's topic and main idea. As seen in question 27, the main purpose of this article is to use historical evidence to provide counterarguments to anti-Stratfordians. A is simply a definition; C is a supporting detail, not a main idea; and D represents an idea of anti-Stratfordians, not the author's opinion.

9. C: Rhetorical question. This requires readers to be familiar with different types of rhetorical devices. A rhetorical question is a question that is asked not to obtain an answer but to encourage readers to more deeply consider an issue.

10. B: By explaining grade school curriculum in Shakespeare's time. This question asks readers to refer to the organizational structure of the article and demonstrate understanding of how the author provides details to support their argument. This particular detail can be found in the second paragraph: "even though he did not attend university, grade school education in Shakespeare's time was actually quite rigorous."

11. A: Busy. This is a vocabulary question that can be answered using context clues. Other sentences in the paragraph describe London as "the most populous city in England" filled with "crowds of people," giving an image of a busy city full of people. *B* is not correct because London was in Shakespeare's home country, not a foreign one. *C* is not mentioned in the passage. *D* is not a good answer choice because the passage describes how London was a popular and important city, probably not an underdeveloped one.

12. D: In Shakespeare's time, glove-makers were not part of the upper class. Anti-Stratfordians doubt Shakespeare's ability because he was not from the upper class; his father was a glove-maker; therefore, in at least this instance, glove-makers were not included in the upper class (this is an example of inductive reasoning, or using two specific pieces of information to draw a more general conclusion).

13. C: It is an example of a play set outside of England. This detail comes from the third paragraph, where the author responds to skeptics who claim that Shakespeare wrote too much about places he never visited, so *Romeo and Juliet* is mentioned as a famous example of a play with a foreign setting. In order to answer this question, readers need to understand the author's main purpose in the third paragraph and how the author uses details to support this purpose. *A* and *D* are not mentioned in the passage, and *B* is clearly not true because the passage mentions more than once that Shakespeare never left England.

14. A: It is possible to learn things from reading rather than from firsthand experience. This inference can be made from the final paragraph, where the author refutes anti-Stratfordian skepticism by pointing out that books about life in Europe could easily circulate throughout London. From this statement, readers can conclude that the author believes it is possible that Shakespeare learned about European culture from books, rather than visiting the continent on his own. *B* is not true because the author believes that Shakespeare contributed to English literature without traveling extensively. Similarly, *C* is not a good answer because the author explains how Shakespeare got his education without university. *D* can also be eliminated because the author describes Shakespeare's genius and clearly Shakespeare is not from Italy.

15. B: A period of time. "Four score and seven years ago" is the equivalent of eighty-seven years, because the word "score" means "twenty." *A* and *C* are incorrect because the context for describing a unit of measurement or a literary movement is lacking. *D* is incorrect because although Lincoln's speech is a cornerstone in political rhetoric, the phrase "Four score and seven years ago" is better narrowed to a period of time.

16. C: The setting of this text is a battlefield in Gettysburg, PA. *A, B,* and *D* are incorrect because the text specifies they are "met on a great battlefield of that war."

17. D: Abraham Lincoln is the former president of the United States, so the correct answer is *D*, "The American Civil War." Though the U.S. was involved in World War I and II, *A* and *C* are incorrect because a civil war specifically means citizens fighting within the same country. *B* is incorrect, as "The War of Spanish Succession" involved Spain, Italy, Germany, and Holland, and not the United States.

18. A: The speech calls on the audience to consider the soldiers who died on the battlefield as ideas to perpetuate freedom so that their deaths would not be in vain. *B* is incorrect because, although they are there to "dedicate a portion of that field," there is no mention in the text of an annual memorial service. *C* is incorrect because there is no charged language in the text, only reverence for the dead. *D* is incorrect because "forget[ting] the lives that were lost" is the opposite of what Lincoln is suggesting.

19. D: Choice *A*, antimetabole, is the repetition of words in a succession. Choice *B*, antiphrasis, is a form of denial of an assertion in a text. Choice *D* is the correct answer; the repetition of the word "people" at the end of the passage. Choice *C*, anaphora, is the repetition that occurs at the beginning of the sentences.

20. A: Choice *A* is correct because Lincoln's intention was to memorialize the soldiers who had fallen as a result of war as well as celebrate those who had put their lives in danger for the sake of their country. Choices *B*, *C*, and *D* are incorrect because Lincoln's speech was supposed to foster a sense of pride among the members of the audience while connecting them to the soldiers' experiences, not to alienate or discourage them.

21. D: The use of "you" could have all of the effects for the reader with the Choices *A*, *B*, and *C*; it could serve to personalize the text, make the passage easier to understand, and cause the reader to empathize with Henrietta Lack's story. However, it doesn't distance the reader from Lack's experiences, thus eliminating Choice *D*.

22. A: Choices *C* and *D* are incorrect because they are disproven in the text. Choice *B* is incorrect because there is no mention of what the best evidence of cell mutation is. The author references Dolly to point the reader to another popular case of DNA research.

23. D: The word "harness" in the text means to duplicate because the scientists' desire is to develop more immortal cells. *A*, "tack," means to pinpoint in place with tacks, which is physically impossible in this context. *B*, "obtain," doesn't logically make sense, because the scientists couldn't obtain traits at this stage in their development. *C*, "couple," is also incorrect, as scientists in this context are more prone to duplicating unique traits than coupling them.

24. D: Choice *D* is correct because the text states that HeLa cells came from a sliver of one of the Henrietta Lack's tumor. Choice *A* and *B* are not mentioned in the text, and Choice *C* is incorrect, as the HeLa cells did not come through DNA testing.

25. D: The discovery of HeLa cells has helped to further the scientific world through *A*, isolating stem cells, *B*, cloning whole animals, and *D*, in vitro fertilization. Choice *D*, separating Siamese twins, is not mentioned in the text.

26. C: The text states that normally developed humans have 46 chromosomes. Originally scientists thought that human cells contained 48 chromosomes, but later a geneticist in Texas proved that incorrect.

27. A: The story is dedicated to telling about the origin of the battery. It doesn't explicitly explain the mechanics of battery operated machines or the far-reaching effects of battery usage, like Choices *B* and *C* suggest. Choice *D* also doesn't work because it does not explicitly encourage readers to take part in new innovations.

28. A: Choices *B* and *D* are incorrect because the text makes no mention of an assessment or a violent encounter. Choice *C* is a possibility; however, Choice *A* is the correct answer because Volta placed things in a particular order to achieve a given result.

29. A: Choice *A*, problem and solution, is the correct answer because the passage details the problem of trying to use electricity to induce muscle contraction and the solution of causing metals to touch instead of muscles, which later lead to the development of the battery.

30. C: The text states that Volta is credited with creating the first battery. Choice *A*, Galvani, had a part in the discovery of the battery because Volta built upon Galvani's previous research. Choice *B*, Pavia, is the university that Volta attended. Choice *D*, Bologna, is the name of the university that Galvani attended.

31. C: The text supports the idea that the term "voltage" has a direct correlation to the fact that Volta is the scientist credited with originally developing batteries. *A* is incorrect because the text does not explain how the researcher died, or that he had failed in any way. *B* is incorrect because information about the researcher's peers is not represented in the text. *D* is incorrect because the text does not divulge the advances of modern researchers.

32. C: The text corroborates the assertion concerning Galvani's belief about the role of animals' life-force in inducing muscle movements. Volta's initial doubt in Galvani's belief led Volta to further the research Galvani had started. *A* is incorrect because it leaves out any information concerning Volta. *B* is incorrect because Volta was not concerned with the intellect of the animals, but rather their ability to contain the "life-force" of electricity. *D* is incorrect because the text does not depict either researcher believing their own theories were the foremost research in the field.

33. C: The text mentions all of the listed properties of minerals except the instance of minerals being organically formed. Objects or substances must be naturally occurring, must be a homogeneous solid, and must have a definite chemical composition in order to be considered a mineral.

34. A: Choice *A* is the correct answer because geology is the study of earth related science. Choice *B* is incorrect because psychology is the study of the mind and behavior. Choice *C* is incorrect because biology is the study of life and living organisms. Choice *D* is incorrect because botany is the study of plants.

35. A: Choice *A* is the correct answer because the prefix "homo" means same. Choice *B* is incorrect because "differing in some areas" would be linked to the root word "hetero," meaning "different" or "other."

36: C: Choice *C* is the correct answer because *-logy* refers to the study of a particular subject matter.

37: C: Choice *C* is the correct answer because the counterargument is necessary to point to the fact that researchers don't always agree with findings. Choices *A* and *B* are incorrect because the counterargument isn't overcomplicated or expressing bias, but simply stating an objective dispute. Choice *D* is incorrect because the counterargument is not used to persuade readers to create a new subsection of minerals.

38. D: Choice *D* is correct because the selection is told from first person but also addresses the reader as "you." *A* is incorrect because while the perspective is told from an "I" perspective, it also addresses the reader by the use of the word "you." *B* is incorrect because just like A, the selection addresses the reader, but also is told from a first person perspective. *C* is incorrect because there are no third-person pronouns in this selection.

39. A: Not only does the article provide examples to disprove a myth, the title also suggests that the article is trying to disprove a myth. Further, the sentence, "But the 'fact' that the majority of your body heat is lost through your head is a lie," and then the subsequent "let me explain," demonstrates the author's intention in disproving a myth. *B* is incorrect because although the selection does compare elephants and anteaters, it does so in order to prove a point, and is not the primary reason that the selection was written. *C* is incorrect because even though the article mentions somebody wearing clothes in the winter, and that doing so could save your life, wearing clothes in the winter is not the primary reason this article was written. *D* is incorrect because the article only mentions that people are gullible once, and makes no further comment on the matter, so this cannot be the primary purpose.

40. B: If the myth is that most of one's body heat is lost through their head, then the fact that heat loss is proportional to surface area exposed is the best evidence that disproves it, since one's head is a great deal less surface area than the rest of the body, making *B* the correct choice. "It is better to wear a shirt than a hat" does not provide evidence that disproves the fact that the head loses more heat than the rest of the body. Thus, *A* is incorrect. *C* is incorrect because gullibility is mentioned only once in this passage and the rest of the article ignores this statement, so clearly it is not the main idea. Finally, *D* is incorrect because though the article mentions that the human chest probably loses the most heat, it is to provide an example of the evidence that heat loss is proportional to surface area exposed, so this is not the main idea of the passage.

41. B: Choice *B* is correct because the author is trying to demonstrate the main idea, which is that heat loss is proportional to surface area, and so they compare two animals with different surface areas to clarify the main point. *A* is incorrect because the author uses elephants and anteaters to prove a point, that heat loss is proportional to surface area, not to express an opinion. *C* is incorrect because though the author does use them to show differences, they do so in order to give examples that prove the above points, so *C* is not the best answer. *D* is incorrect because there is no language to indicate favoritism between the two animals.

42. C: Since there is an opinion presented along with a fact, *C* is the correct answer. *A* is incorrect—"Not only would you look stupid," is an opinion because there is no way to prove that somebody would look stupid by not wearing a shirt in the cold, even if that may be a popular opinion. However, this opinion is sandwiched inside a factual statement. *B* is incorrect because again, this is a factual statement, but it has been editorialized by interjecting an opinion. Because of the presence of both a fact and an opinion, *D* is the opposite of the correct answer.

43. C: Because of the way that the author addresses the reader, and also the colloquial language that the author uses (i.e., "let me explain," "so," "well," didn't," "you would look stupid," etc.), *C* is the best answer because it has a much more casual tone than the usual informative article. Choice *A* may be a tempting choice because the author says the "fact" that most of one's heat is lost through their head is a "lie," and that someone who does not wear a shirt in the cold looks stupid, but it only happens twice within all the diction of the passage and it does not give an overall tone of harshness. *B* is incorrect because again, while not necessarily nice, the language does not carry an angry charge. The author is clearly not indifferent to the subject because of the passionate language that they use, so *D* is incorrect.

44. A: The author gives logical examples and reason in order to prove that most of one's heat is not lost through their head, therefore *A* is correct. *B* is incorrect because there is not much emotionally charged language in this selection, and even the small amount present is greatly outnumbered by the facts and evidence. *C* is incorrect because there is no mention of ethics or morals in this selection. *D* is incorrect because the author never qualifies themselves as someone who has the authority to be writing on this topic.

45. C: Choice *C* is correct because it contains factual evidence used to disprove a theory, and has no persuasive intent. *A* is incorrect because the selection does not follow a series of events or plot of any kind, nor does it have any elements of a narrative (plot, characters, setting, and theme). *B* is incorrect because the article does not attempt to persuade the reader that this is true; the author simply says that it is true, and is not asking the reader to take a stance on it. Finally, there are not any obvious descriptions within the passage, so *D* is incorrect.

46. B: Choice *B* is correct because since the primary purpose of the article is to provide evidence to disprove the myth that most of a person's heat is lost through their head, then each part of the body losing heat in proportion to its surface area is the best evidence to disprove the myth. *A* is incorrect because again, gullibility is not a main contributor to this article, but it may be common to see questions on the test that give the same wrong answer in order to try and trick the test taker. Choice *C* only suggests what you should do with this information; it is not the primary evidence itself. Choice *D*, while tempting, is actually not evidence. It does not give any reason for why it is a lie; it simply states that it is. Evidence is factual information that supports a claim.

Vocabulary

1. C: Contralateral. As a prefix, *contra-* means opposite or against. In this case, *contralateral* means on the opposite side of the body.

2. A: Enlarged or expanded. A *distended* stomach or other organ is bloated or swollen because of internal pressure.

3. B: Precipitously. *Concisely* means in a few words or efficiently worded, *contingently* refers to something that will occur only if something else happens first, and *preemptively* means something taken as a precaution or measure against an anticipated risk or problem, often as a way to try and prevent it.

4. A: Patent. In a medical context, a *patent* vessel is unobstructed and open. An atherosclerotic vessel with deposited plaques would probably not be *patent*.

5. D: Absence of menstruation. The prefix *a-* means "not" or "anti." *Menses* is the menstrual cycle, and the suffix *-rhea* means "flow." Therefore, *amenorrhea* is the absence of a menstrual period.

6. C: Present but not active or visible. A *latent* disease is present but not detectable in a symptomatic way. It may be dormant, but has to potential to become symptomatic in the future with discernable manifestations for the patient.

7. C: Overt. *Obsolete* means outdated or no longer produced or used, *covert* means not outwardly acknowledged or shown, and to *collude* is to conspire.

8. A: Difficulty breathing. The prefix *dys-* means dysfunctional or abnormal. *-Pnea* in a medical context refers to respiration and breathing. Sleep apnea is a breathing disorder that can occur during sleep.

9. B: Sudden or rapid onset. An *acute* illness is the opposite of a *chronic* one, which is a disease that the patient has had for a long time. A sinus infection is an acute illness, while multiple sclerosis is a chronic one.

10. D: Virulent. *Patent* means open, *innocuous* means harmless, and *latent* means dormant.

11. C: Undesirable. An adverse reaction to a medication is an undesirable side effect or consequence of taking the drug.

12. B: Insidious. *Precipitous* means rapid or steep, *incipient* means emergent or at an initial state, and *paroxysmal* means a sudden intensification or recurrence of symptoms, as in a paroxysmal attack of a muscle spasm in the lumbar spine.

13. A: Lack of urine output. Again, the prefixes *a-* or *an-* mean "without" or "not," and *-uria* refers to urine.

14. C: Proximal. *Distal* is the opposite of proximal. Distal means further from the trunk (usually down an extremity).

15. C: Impervious. *Impotent,* in the medical context, means unable to achieve sexual arousal (for a man). In general, the word means powerless. *Hygienic* means sanitary. *Impending* means imminent.

16. B: Origin or cause. Some diseases have an unknown etiology.

17. D: Endogenous. The prefix *endo-* means "within" or "containing," and *-genous* means originating in or producing. The prefix *exo-* means the "outside."

18. A: Febrile. *Futile* means pointless, *libel* is printed defamation of someone's character, and *liable* means responsible, especially in a legal sense.

19. A: Multiplied or increased in number. Given the right conditions, bacterial cells *proliferate* rapidly.

20. B: A fluid's thickness or resistance to flow. A viscous fluid is in contrast to a runny one. For example, honey is more viscous than water.

21. B: Supine. *Prone* is the position on one's stomach.

22. C: Environment. For example, the internal *milieu* usually refers to interstitial fluid.

23. D: Abnormal. *Overt* means outwardly demonstrative, *grave* means severe or serious, and *radical* means revolutionary or progressive.

24. B: Laceration. An *incision* is a more precise cut, as in one made by a surgeon using a scalpel during surgery. A *contusion* is a bruise and an *avulsion* is a type of fracture where a piece of the bone is ripped off.

25. C: Relating to the kidney. The renal blood vessels serve the kidneys.

26. A: Debridement. An *arthroscopy* is a type of surgical procedure on a joint using a camera and small scope, *distension* is swelling or bloating, and a *laparoscopy* is a surgical procedure that involves the insertion of a fiberoptic instrument.

27. D: Sort based on problem severity. Patients entering the ER need to be triaged so that they are treated in order of urgency.

28. D: Predisposed. *Predisposed* means inclined to a specific condition or action.

29. B: Dilate. To *dilute* is to make a solution less concentrated, *occlude* means to block or obstruct, and *distill* means to purify a liquid or to extract the most important aspects or meaning of something.

30. C: Lethargic. *Indolent* can also mean lazy or aversive to activity.

31. D: Veins. Arteries bring blood from the heart to the tissues and veins return the blood to the heart from the tissues.

32. D: Inside the cheek. An example of a medication with a buccal route of administration is nitroglycerine in the treatment of angina.

33. B: Teacher. *Pupil* means student.

34. A: To cough out phlegm. Someone with pneumonia may *expectorate* in the sink.

35. A: Home. Like the word *reside,* which means to inhabit, a *residence* is where someone lives.

36. D: To *relinquish* something is to give up claim to it. For example, a spouse trying to be more considerate may relinquish the TV remote so that his or her partner can choose a show.

37. C: To *germinate* is to develop or come into existence. A novel marketing idea might germinate at a business lunch. In a botany context, it also means to sprout or bud.

38. A: Insurance. *Indemnity* is an insurance or other security or safeguard against a financial burden or loss.

39. C: Unrestrained. *Stagnant* means still or unchanging, like a body of water with no active flow.

40. D: Threatening. Choices *B* and *C, promising* and *auspicious,* are antonyms of *ominous.*

41. A: Hypoglycemia. *Hypo-* means "below" or "beneath," and *glycemia* comes from glucose, so it refers to blood sugar.

42. A: Watched. To *observe* is to watch or examine with one's eyes.

43. C: Somnolent. Someone *comatose* is unresponsive to stimuli. Someone *delirious* is either ecstatic or mentally disturbed and seeing illusions.

44. B: Hemoptysis. The suffix *-ptysis* means spitting of matter.

45. D: Swell. A tissue that is *engorged* is swollen with fluid. For example, a new mom will have breasts engorged with milk to nurture her baby.

46. A: Bereavement. *Disposition* is someone's personality or affect, *depression* is a state of a low mood, and *belligerent* means aggressive and hostile.

47. C: Polydipsia. *Poly-* means "many" or "multiple" and the suffix *-dipsia* refers to thrist.

48. C: Able to feel or perceive. A *sentient* being is living and able to perceive or feel something and respond.

49. C: Relating to digestion. *Peptic* comes from *pepsin,* which is a stomach enzyme that helps degrade proteins.

50. A: Isometric. The prefix *iso-* means "same" and *-metric* refers to length.

Grammar

1. D: To begin, *of* is not required here. *Apprenticeship* is also more appropriate in this context than *apprentice opportunities, apprentice* describes an individual in an apprenticeship, not an apprenticeship itself. Both of these changes are needed, making (*D*) the correct answer.

2. D: To begin, the selected sentence is a run-on, and displays discombobulated information. Thus, the sentence does need revision, making (*A*) wrong. The main objective of the selected section of the passage is to communicate that many positions (*positions* is a more suitable term than *offices*, as well) require a PE license, which is gained by scoring well on the FE and PE assessments. This must be the primary focus of the revision. It is necessary to break the sentence into two, to avoid a run-on. Choice *B* fixes the run-on aspect, but the sentence is indirect and awkward in construction. It takes too long to establish the importance of the PE license. Choice *C* is wrong for the same reason and it is a run on. Choice *D* is correct because it breaks the section into coherent sentences and emphasizes the main point the author is trying to communicate: the PE license is required for some higher positions, it's obtained by scoring well on the two standardized assessments, and college and experience can be used to prepare for the assessments in order to gain the certification.

3. C: *Allows* is inappropriate because it does not stress what those in the position of aircraft engineers actually need to be able to do. *Requires* is the only alternative that fits because it actually describes necessary skills of the job.

4. A: The correct response is (*A*) because this statement's intent is to give examples as to how aircraft engineers apply mathematical equations and scientific processes towards aeronautical and aerospace issues and/or inventions. The answer is not "therefore" (*B*) or "furthermore" (*D*) because no causality is being made between ideas. Two items are neither being compared nor contrasted, so "however" (*C*) is also not the correct answer.

5. A: No change is required. The comma is properly placed after the introductory phrase "In May of 2015." Choice *B* is missing the word "in." Choice *C* does not separate the introductory phrase from the rest of the sentence. Choice *D* places an extra, and unnecessary, comma prior to 2015.

6. A: The word "conversely" best demonstrates the opposite sentiments in this passage. Choice *B* is incorrect because it denotes agreement with the previous statement. Choice *C* is incorrect because the sentiment is not restated, but opposed. Choice *D* is incorrect because the previous statement is not a cause for the sentence in question.

7. A: Choice *A* is the correct answer because the projections are taking place in the present, even though they are making reference to a future date.

8. A: No change is needed. Choices *B* and *C* utilize incorrect comma placements. Choice *D* utilizes an incorrect verb tense (responding).

9. C: All of the choices except (*C*) go with the flow of the original underlined portion of the sentence and communicate the same idea. Choice *C,* however, does not take into account the rest of the sentence and therefore, becomes awkward and incorrect.

10. B: Although "diverging" means to separate from the main route and go in a different direction, it is used awkwardly and unconventionally in this sentence. Therefore, Choice *A* is not the answer. Choice *B* is the correct answer because it implies that the passengers distracted the terrorists, which caused a change in the plane's direction. "Converging" (*C*) is incorrect because it implies that the plane met another in a central location. Although the passengers may have distracted the terrorists, they did not distract the plane. Therefore, Choice *D* is incorrect.

11. A: Choice *C* can be eliminated because creating a new sentence with *not* is grammatically incorrect and it throws off the rest of the sentence. Choice *B* is wrong because a comma is definitely needed after *devastation* in the sentence. Choice *D* is also incorrect because "while" is a poor substitute for "although". *Although* in this context is meant to show contradiction with the idea that floods are associated with devastation. Therefore, none of these choices would be suitable revisions because the original was correct: NO CHANGE, Choice *A,* is the correct answer.

12. A: While (*B*) isn't necessarily wrong, it lacks the direct nature that the original sentence has. Also by breaking up the sentences like this, the reader becomes confused because the connection between the Taliban's defeat and ongoing war is now separated by a second sentence that is not necessary. Choice *C* corrects this problem but the fluidity of the sentence is marred because of the awkward construction of the first sentence. Choice *D* begins well, but lacks the use of *was* before overthrown, which discombobulates the sentence. While *yet* provides an adequate transition for the next sentence, the term *however* is more appropriate. Thus, the original structure of the two sentences is correct, making Choice *A,* NO CHANGE, the correct answer.

13. A: The comma after *result* is necessary for the sentence structure, making it an imperative component. The original sentence is correct, making Choice *A* correct. For the reason just listed, Choice *B* is incorrect because it lacks the crucial comma that introduces a new idea. Choice *C* is incorrect because a colon is unnecessary, and Choice *D* is wrong because the addition of "of" is both unnecessary and incorrect when applied to the rest of the sentence.

14. A: No change is needed: Choice *A*. The list of events accomplished by Hampton is short enough that each item in the list can be separated by a comma. Choice *B* is incorrect. Although a colon can be used to introduce a list of items, it is not a conventional choice for separating items within a series. Semicolons are used to separate at least three items in a series that have an internal comma. Semicolons can also be used to separate clauses in a sentence that contain internal commas intended for clarification purposes. Neither of the two latter uses of semicolons is required in the example sentence. Therefore, Choice *C* is incorrect. Choice *D* is incorrect because a dash is not a conventional choice for punctuating items in a series.

15. A: To *project* means to anticipate or forecast. This goes very well with the sentence because it describes how new technology is trying to estimate flood activity in order to prevent damage and save lives. "Project" in this case needs to be assisted by "to" in order to function in the sentence. Therefore, Choice *A* is correct. Choices *B* and *D* are the incorrect tenses. Choice *C* is also wrong because it lacks *to*.

16. B: The order of the original sentence suggests that the floor plans that were provided to the FBI by O'Neal enabled the FBI to identify the exact location of Hampton's bed. This syntax is maintained in Choice *B*. Therefore, Choice *B* is correct, which makes Choice *A* incorrect. Choice *C* is incorrect because the sentence's word order conveys the meaning that O'Neal provided the FBI with Hampton's bed as well as the floor plans. Choice *D* is incorrect because it implies that it was the location of the bed that provided the FBI with the headquarters' floor plans.

17. D: Again, the objective for questions like this is to determine if a revision is possible within the choices and if it can adhere to the specific criteria of the question; in this case, we want the sentence to maintain the original meaning while being more concise, or shorter. Choice *B* can be eliminated. The meaning of the original sentence is split into two distinct sentences. The second of the two sentences is also incorrectly constructed. Choice *C* is very intriguing but there is a jumble of verbs present in: "Flooding occurs slowly or rapidly submerging" that it makes the sentence awkward and difficult to understand without the use of a comma after *rapidly*, making it a poor construction. Choice *C* is wrong. Choice *D* is certainly more concise and it is correctly phrased; it communicates the meaning message that flooding can overtake great lengths of land either slowly or very fast. The use of "Vast areas of land" infers that smaller regions or small areas can flood just as well. Thus, Choice *D* is a good revision that maintains the meaning of the original sentence while being concise and more direct. This rules out Choice *A* in the process.

18. B: In this sentence, the word *ocean* does not require an *s* after it to make it plural because "ocean levels" is plural. Therefore (*A*) and (*C*) are incorrect. Because the passage is referring to multiple – if not all ocean levels – *ocean* does not require an apostrophe (*'s*) because that would indicate that only one ocean is the focus, which is not the case. Choice *D* does not fit well into the sentence and, once again, we see that *ocean* has an *s* after it. This leaves Choice *B,* which correctly completes the sentence and maintains the intended meaning.

19. A: Choice *A* uses incorrect subject-verb agreement because the indefinite pronoun *neither* is singular and must use the singular verb form *is*. The pronoun *both* is plural and uses the plural verb form of *are*. The pronoun *any* can be either singular or plural. In this example, it is used as a plural, so the plural verb form *are* is used. The pronoun *each* is singular and uses the singular verb form *is*.

20. B: Choice *B* is correct because the pronouns *he* and *I* are in the subjective case. *He* and *I* are the subjects of the verb *like* in the independent clause of the sentence. Choice *A, C,* and *D* are incorrect because they all contain at least one objective pronoun (*me* and *him*). Objective pronouns should not be used as the subject of the sentence, but rather, they should come as an object of a verb. To test for correct pronoun usage, try reading the pronouns as if they were the only pronoun in the sentence. For example, *he* and *me* may appear to be the correct answer choices, but try reading them as the only pronoun.

He like[s] to go fishing…

Me like to go fishing…

When looked at that way, *me* is an obviously incorrect choice.

21. D: The object pronouns *her* and *me* act as the indirect objects of the sentence. If *me* is in a series of object pronouns, it should always come last in the series. Choice *A* is incorrect because it uses subject pronouns *she* and *I*. Choice *B* is incorrect because it uses the subject pronoun *she*. Choice *C* uses the correct object pronouns, but they are in the wrong order.

22. A: Slang refers to non-standard expressions that are not used in elevated speech and writing. Slang tends to be specific to one group or time period and is commonly used within groups of young people during their conversations with each other. Jargon refers to the language used in a specialized field. The vernacular is the native language of a local area, and a dialect is one form of a language in a certain region. Thus, *B, C,* and *D* are incorrect.

23. D: Colloquial language is that which is used conversationally or informally, in contrast to professional or academic language. While *ain't* is common in conversational English, it is a non-standard expression in academic writing. For college-bound students, high school should introduce them to the expectations of a college classroom, so *B* is not the best answer. Teachers should also avoid placing moral or social value on certain patterns of speech. Rather than teaching students that their familiar speech patterns are bad, teachers should help students learn when and how to use appropriate forms of expression, so *C* is wrong. *Ain't* is in the dictionary, so *A* is incorrect, both in the reason for counseling and in the factual sense.

24. C: A complex sentence joins an independent or main clause with a dependent or subordinate clause. In this case, the main clause is "The restaurant is unconventional." This is a clause with one subject-verb combination that can stand alone as a grammatically-complete sentence. The dependent clause is "because it serves both Chicago style pizza and New York style pizza." This clause begins with the subordinating conjunction *because* and also consists of only one subject-verb combination. *A* is incorrect because a simple sentence consists of only one verb-subject combination—one independent clause. *B* is incorrect because a compound sentence contains two independent clauses connected by a conjunction. *D* is incorrect because a complex-compound sentence consists of two or more independent clauses and one or more dependent clauses.

25. A: Parallelism refers to consistent use of sentence structure or word form. In this case, the list within the sentence does not utilize parallelism; three of the verbs appear in their base form—*travel*, *take*, and *eat*—but one appears as a gerund—*going*. A parallel version of this sentence would be "This summer, I'm planning to travel to Italy, take a Mediterranean cruise, go to Pompeii, and eat a lot of Italian food." *B* is incorrect because this description is a complete sentence. *C* is incorrect as a misplaced modifier is a modifier that is not located appropriately in relation to the word or words they modify. *D* is incorrect because subject-verb agreement refers to the appropriate conjugation of a verb in relation to its subject.

26. C: In this sentence, the modifier is the phrase "Forgetting that he was supposed to meet his girlfriend for dinner." This phrase offers information about Fred's actions, but the noun that immediately follows it is Anita, creating some confusion about the "do-er" of the phrase. A more appropriate sentence arrangement would be "Forgetting that he was supposed to meet his girlfriend for dinner, Fred made Anita mad when he showed up late." *A* is incorrect as parallelism refers to the consistent use of sentence structure and verb tense, and this sentence is appropriately consistent. *B* is incorrect as a run-on sentence does not contain appropriate punctuation for the number of independent clauses presented, which is not true of this description. *D* is incorrect because subject-verb agreement refers to the appropriate conjugation of a verb relative to the subject, and all verbs have been properly conjugated.

27. B: A comma splice occurs when a comma is used to join two independent clauses together without the additional use of an appropriate conjunction. One way to remedy this problem is to replace the comma with a semicolon. Another solution is to add a conjunction: "Some workers use all their sick leave, but other workers cash out their leave." *A* is incorrect as parallelism refers to the consistent use of sentence structure and verb tense; all tenses and structures in this sentence are consistent. *C* is incorrect because a sentence fragment is a phrase or clause that cannot stand alone—this sentence contains two independent clauses. *D* is incorrect because subject-verb agreement refers to the proper conjugation of a verb relative to the subject, and all verbs have been properly conjugated.

28. D: The problem in the original passage is that the second sentence is a dependent clause that cannot stand alone as a sentence; it must be attached to the main clause found in the first sentence. Because the main clause comes first, it does not need to be separated by a comma. However, if the dependent clause came first, then a comma would be necessary, which is why Choice *C* is incorrect. *A* and *B* also insert unnecessary commas into the sentence.

29. A: A noun refers to a person, place, thing, or idea. Although the word *approach* can also be used as a verb, in the sentence it functions as a noun within the noun phrase "a fresh approach," so *B* is incorrect. An adverb is a word or phrase that provides additional information of the verb, but because the verb is *need* and not *approach*, then *C* is false. An adjective is a word that describes a noun, used here as the word *fresh*, but it is not the noun itself. Thus, *D* is also incorrect.

30. D: An adjective modifies a noun, answering the question "Which one?" or "What kind?" In this sentence, the word *exhaustive* is an adjective that modifies the noun *investigation*. Another clue that this word is an adjective is the suffix *–ive*, which means "having the quality of." The noun in this sentence is *investigators*; therefore, *A* is incorrect. The verb in this sentence is *conducted* because this was the action taken by the subject *the investigators*; therefore, *B* is incorrect. *C* is incorrect because an adverb is a word or phrase that provides additional information about the verb, expressing how, when, where, or in what manner.

31. B: In this case, the phrase functions as an adverb modifying the verb *report*, so *B* is the correct answer. "To the student center" does not consist of a subject-verb combination, so it is not a clause; thus, Choices *A* and *C* can be eliminated. This group of words is a phrase. Phrases are classified by either the controlling word in the phrase or its function in the sentence. *D* is incorrect because a noun phrase is a series of words that describe or modify a noun.

32. D: In this sentence, the first answer choice requires a noun meaning *impact* or *influence*, so *effect* is the correct answer. For the second answer choice, the sentence is drawing a comparison. *Than* shows a comparative relationship whereas *then* shows sequence or consequence. *A* and *C* can be eliminated because they contain the choice *then*. *B* is incorrect because *affect* is a verb while this sentence requires a noun.

33. D: Since the sentence contains two independent clauses and a dependent clause, the sentence is categorized as compound-complex:

> Independent clause: *I accepted the change of seasons*

> Independent clause: *I started to appreciate the fall*

> Dependent clause: *Although I wished it were summer*

34. D: Students can use context clues to make a careful guess about the meaning of unfamiliar words. Although all of the words in a sentence can help contribute to the overall sentence, in this case, the adjective that pairs with *ubiquitous* gives the most important hint to the student—cars were first *rare*, but now they are *ubiquitous*. The inversion of *rare* is what gives meaning to the rest of the sentence and *ubiquitous* means "existing everywhere" or "not rare." *A* is incorrect because *ago* only indicates a time frame. *B* is incorrect because *cars* does not indicate a contrasting relationship to the word *ubiquitous* to provide a good context clue. *C* is incorrect because it also only indicates a time frame, but used together with *rare*, it provides the contrasting relationship needed to identify the meaning of the unknown word.

35. B: Proper nouns are specific. *Statue of Liberty* is a proper noun and specifies exactly which statue is being discussed. Choice *A* is incorrect because the word *people* is a common noun and it is only capitalized because it is at the beginning of the sentence. Choice *C* is incorrect. The word *awesome* is an adjective describing the sight. Choice *D* is incorrect. The word *sight* is a common noun. A clue to eliminate answer choices *C* and *D* is that they were not capitalized. Proper nouns are always capitalized.

36. B: The word *kittens* is plural, meaning more than one kitten. Choice *A* is incorrect. The word *kitten* is singular. Choice *B* is incorrect. The word *girl's* is a singular possessive form. The girl is making the choice. There is only one girl involved. Choice *C* is incorrect. The word *choice* is a singular noun. The girl has only one choice to make. The word *litter* in this sentence is a collective plural noun meaning a group of kittens.

37. C: The word *who* in the sentence is a subjective interrogative pronoun and the sentence needed a subject that begins a question. Choice *A* is incorrect. The word *whose* is a possessive pronoun and it is not being asked who owns the flowers. Choice *B* is incorrect. The word *whom* is always an objective pronoun—never a subjective one; a subjective pronoun is needed in this sentence. Choice *D* is incorrect. The word *who've* is a contraction of the words *who* and *have*. We would not say, *"Who have ordered the flowers?"*

38. D: The word *its* in the sentence is the singular possessive form of the pronoun that stands in place for the word *giraffe's.* There is one baby that belongs to one giraffe. Choice *A* is incorrect. It is a contraction of the words *it* and *is.* You would not say, *"The giraffe nudged it is baby."* Choice *B* is incorrect. We do not know the gender of the giraffe and if it was female the proper word would be *her* baby not *hers* baby. Choice *C* is incorrect. The word *their* is a plural possessive pronoun and we need a singular possessive pronoun because there is only one giraffe doing the nudging.

39. B: The word *several* stands in for a plural noun at the beginning of the sentence, such as the noun *people.* It is also an indefinite pronoun because the number of people, for example, is not defined. Choice *A* is incorrect. The pronoun is plural not singular. It indicates more than one person. We can tell because the sentence works with the plural word *are* for the verb; substituting the singular word *is* would not make sense. We wouldn't say, *"Several is laughing loudly on the bus."* Choice *C* is incorrect. *Several* is the subject of the sentence. Therefore, it is a subjective pronoun not an objective one. Choice *D* is incorrect. The word *several* does not modify a noun in the sentence. If the sentence said, *"Several people are laughing loudly on the bus,"* then the word *several* would be an indefinite adjective modifying the word *people.*

40. A: The word *delectable* is an adjective modifying the noun *meal* in the sentence. It answers the question: *"What kind of meal?"* Choice *B* is incorrect. The word *connoisseur* is a noun that is the subject of the sentence. Choice *C* is incorrect. The word *slowly* is an adverb telling how the subject enjoyed the meal. Choice *D* is incorrect. The word *enjoyed* is the past-tense verb in the sentence telling us what action the subject had taken.

41. B: The word *by* is a positional preposition telling where we are in relation to the water. The word *near* is also a positional preposition telling where *we* are in relation to the lake. The word *before* is a time preposition telling when in relation to the time of day, dawn. Choice *A* is incorrect because *went* and *to see* are both verbs and *pretty* is an adjective modifying the word *sunrise.* Choice *C* is incorrect because *water, lake, dawn,* and *sunrise* are all nouns in the sentence. Choice *D* is incorrect because the word *we* is a pronoun, the word *down* is an adverb modifying the verb *went,* the word *the* is an article, and the word *pretty* is an adjective modifying *sunrise.*

42. B: The word *well* at the beginning of the sentence is set apart from the rest of the sentence with a comma and is a mild interjection. Choice *A* is incorrect. The word *goodness* at the end of the sentence is a noun. It is the idea/state of being for the cookie. Choice *C* is incorrect. It is an interrogative sentence and all of the words in the sentence can be identified as other parts of speech. *Can't* is a contraction of the word cannot and it works with the word *see* as the verb in the sentence. The word *you* is a pronoun; the word *that* is an adjective modifying the word *cookie*; *cookie* is a noun; *is* is another verb; and *broken* is an adjective modifying the word *cookie*. Choice *D* is incorrect because the exclamation mark at the end of the sentence is not there to set apart an interjection. Rather, it is there to punctuate the exclamatory sentence.

43. C: The simple subject is *bike* and its modifiers *heaviest* and *green* are included to form the complete subject. Choice *A* is incorrect because *bike* is the simple subject. Choice *B* is incorrect because it includes only one of the modifiers (*green*) of the word *bike*. Choice *D* is incorrect because *is mine* is the predicate of the sentence, not the subject.

44. D: The subject of the sentence is *my house;* therefore the rest of the sentence is the predicate. Choice *A* is incorrect because *my house* is the subject, not the predicate. Choice *B* is incorrect because *is the yellow one* is only part of the predicate, but the sentence does not end there. Choice *C* is incorrect because *at the end of the street* is only a portion of the predicate.

45. B: The *kitten* is a singular subject and so the singular verb *pounces* should be used instead of *pounce*. Choice *A* is incorrect because the plural subject *kittens* agrees with the plural verb *show*. Choice *C* is incorrect because the singular subject *kitten* agrees with the singular verb *eats*. Choice *D* is incorrect because the singular subject *kitten* agrees with the singular verb *snuggles*.

46. C: *Her mother* is to whom Calysta brought the lamp. Choice *A* is incorrect because *stained-glass lamp* is the direct object of the sentence. Choice *B* is incorrect because *brought* is the verb. Choice *D* is incorrect because *beautiful* is an adjective modifying the noun *lamp*.

47. C: *They're* (they are) on *their* (possessive) way to New Jersey but *they're* (they are) not *there* (location) yet. This sentence makes sense. Choice *A* is incorrect because the sentence does not make sense. After the word *but* should be the word *they're* (they are). Choice *B* is incorrect because the sentence should begin with *they're* (they are) instead of *their* (possessive). Choice *D* is incorrect because after the word *not* should be *there* (location) instead of *their* (possessive).

48. D: *For the longest time* is an introductory prepositional phrase beginning with the preposition *for* and all the modifiers for the word *time*. Choice *A* is incorrect because it includes the past-tense verb *have wanted* creating a clause. Choice *B* is incorrect because it includes the verb *wanted* and the infinitive *to learn*. Choice *C* is incorrect because it includes the verb *learn* and the infinitive *to skate*.

49. B: *The weight of the world was on his shoulders* and *he took a long walk* are both independent clauses connected with a comma and a coordinating conjunction. Choice *A* is incorrect because there are two independent clauses and a simple sentence has only one independent clause. Choice *C* is incorrect because the sentence has no dependent clauses and a complex sentence needs at least one dependent clause. Choice *D* is incorrect because, although there are two independent clauses, there are no dependent clauses and a compound-complex sentence will have at least two independent clauses and at least one dependent clause.

50. A: *"The last thing she wanted to do was see the Eiffel Tower before the flight,"* has only one independent clause and no dependent clauses therefore it is a simple sentence. Choice *B* is incorrect because the sentence has only one independent clause. *The last thing she wanted to do* is a gerund phrase serving as the noun subject of the sentence, therefore it is not an independent clause. Choice *C* is incorrect because the sentence has no dependent clauses therefore it cannot be a complex sentence.

Choice *D* is incorrect because the sentence has only one independent clause and no dependent clauses. A compound-complex sentence needs at least two independent clauses and at least one dependent clause.

Biology

1. D: The theory that certain physical and behavioral traits give a species an evolutionary advantage is called natural selection. Charles Darwin developed the theory of natural selection that explains the evolutionary process. He postulated that heritable genetic differences could aid an organism's chance of survival in its environment. The organisms with favorable traits pass genes to their offspring, and because they have more reproductive success than those that do not contain the adaptation, the favorable gene spreads throughout the population. Those that do not contain the adaptation often extinguish; thus, their genes are not passed on. In this way, nature "selects" for the organisms that have more fitness in their environment. Birds with bright colored feathers and cacti with spines are examples of "fit" organisms.

2. D: Water's unique properties are due to intermolecular hydrogen bonding. These forces make water molecules "stick" to one another, which explains why water has unusually high cohesion and adhesion (sticking to each other and sticking to other surfaces). Cohesion can be seen in beads of dew. Adhesion can be seen when water sticks to the sides of a graduated cylinder to form a meniscus. The stickiness to neighboring molecules also increases surface tension, providing a very thin film that light things cannot penetrate, which is observed when leaves float in swimming pools. Water has a low freezing point, not a high freezing point, due to the fact that molecules have to have a very low kinetic energy to arrange themselves in the lattice-like structure found in ice, its solid form.

3. A: Catabolic reactions release energy and are exothermic. Catabolism breaks down complex molecules into simpler molecules. Anabolic reactions are just the opposite—they absorb energy in order to form complex molecules from simpler ones. Proteins, carbohydrates (polysaccharides), lipids, and nucleic acids are complex organic molecules synthesized by anabolic metabolism. The monomers of these organic compounds are amino acids, monosaccharides, triglycerides, and nucleotides.

4. C: Metabolic reactions utilize enzymes to decrease their activation energy. Enzymes that drive these reactions are protein catalysts. Their mechanism is sometimes referred to as the "lock-and-key" model. "Lock and key" references the fact that enzymes have exact specificity with their substrate (reactant) like a lock does to a key. The substrate binds to the enzyme snugly, the enzyme facilitates the reaction, and then product is formed while the enzyme is unchanged and ready to be reused.

5. B: The structure exclusively found in eukaryotic cells is the nucleus. Animal, plant, fungi, and protist cells are all eukaryotic. DNA is contained within the nucleus of eukaryotic cells, and they also have membrane-bound organelles that perform complex intracellular metabolic activities. Prokaryotic cells (archae and bacteria) do not have a nucleus or other membrane-bound organelles and are less complex than eukaryotic cells.

6. A:. The Golgi complex, also known as the Golgi apparatus, is not found in the nucleus. Chromosomes, the nucleolus, and chromatin are all found within the nucleus of the cell. The Golgi apparatus is found in the cytoplasm and is responsible for protein maturation, the process of proteins folding into their secondary, tertiary, and quaternary configurations. The structure appears folded in membranous layers and is easily visible with microscopy. The Golgi apparatus packages proteins in vesicles for export out of the cell or to their cellular destination.

7. B: The cell structure responsible for cellular storage, digestion, and waste removal is the lysosome. Lysosomes are like recycle bins. They are filled with digestive enzymes that facilitate catabolic reactions to regenerate monomers.

8. B: The mitochondria are cellular energy generators and the "powerhouses" of the cell. They provide cellular energy in the form of adenosine triphosphate (ATP). This process, called aerobic respiration, uses oxygen plus sugars, proteins, and fats to produce ATP, carbon dioxide, and water. Mitochondria contain their own DNA and ribosomes, which is significant because according to endosymbiotic theory, these structures provide evidence that they used to be independently-functioning prokaryotes.

9. B: Plastids are the photosynthesizing organelles of plants that are not found in animal cells. Plants have the ability to generate their own sugars through photosynthesis, a process where they use pigments to capture the sun's light energy. Chloroplasts are the most prevalent plastid, and chlorophyll is the light-absorbing pigment that absorbs all energy carried in photons except that of green light. This explains why the photosynthesizing parts of plants, predominantly leaves, appear green.

10. B: Diffusion and osmosis are examples of passive transport. Unlike active transport, passive transport does not require cellular energy. Diffusion is the movement of particles, such as ions, nutrients, or waste, from high concentration to low. Osmosis is the spontaneous movement of water from an area of high concentration to one of low concentration. Facilitated diffusion is another type of passive transport where particles move from high concentration to low concentration via a protein channel.

11. B: Phenotypes are observable traits, such as eye color, hair color, blood type, etc. They can also be biochemical or have physiological or behavioral traits. A genotype is the collective gene representation of an individual, whether the genes are expressed or not. Alleles are different forms of the same gene that code for specific traits, like blue eyes or brown eyes. In simple genetics, there are two forms of a gene: dominant and recessive. More complex genetics involves co-dominant, multiple alleles and sex-linked genes. The other answer choices are incorrect because gender is determined by the presence of an entire chromosome, the Y chromosome, and a karyotype is an image of all of individual's chromosomes.

12. D: Reproductive cells are referred to as gametes: egg (female) and sperm (male). These cells have only 1 set of 23 chromosomes and are haploid so that when they combine during fertilization, the zygote has the correct diploid number, 46. Reproductive cell division is called meiosis, which is different from mitosis, the type of division process for body (somatic) cells.

13. A: The process of cell division in somatic is mitosis. In interphase, which precedes mitosis, cells prepare for division by copying their DNA. Once mitotic machinery has been assembled in interphase, mitosis occurs, which has four distinct phases: prophase, metaphase, anaphase, and telophase, followed by cytokinesis, which is the final splitting of the cytoplasm. The two diploid daughter cells are genetically identical to the parent cell.

14. A: It is the genetic code. Choice *B* is incorrect because DNA does not provide energy—that's the job of carbohydrates and glucose. Choice *C* is incorrect because DNA is double-stranded. Because Choices *B* and *C* are incorrect, Choice *D*, all of the above, is incorrect.

15. D: Glucose exits. The stomata are pores at the bottom of the leaf, and carbon dioxide enters (it is a reactant for photosynthesis) and oxygen exits (it is a product for photosynthesis), so Choices *A* and *C* are correct. Water exits through the stomata in the process of transpiration, so Choice *B* is correct as well.

Glucose is the sugar that is either broken down by the plant for its own energy usage or eaten by other organisms for energy.

16. A: An alteration in the normal gene sequence is called a DNA point mutation. Mutations can be harmful, neutral, or even beneficial. Sometimes, as seen in natural selection, a genetic mutation can improve fitness, providing an adaptation that will aid in survival. DNA mutations can happen as a result of environmental damage, for example, from radiation or chemicals. Mutations can also happen during cell replication, as a result of incorrect pairing of complementary nucleotides by DNA polymerase. There are also chromosomal mutations as well, where entire segments of chromosomes can be deleted, inverted, duplicated, or sent or received from a different chromosome.

17. B: 50%. According to the Punnett square, the child has a 2 out of 4 chance of having A-type blood, since the dominant allele I^A is present in two of the four possible offspring. The O-type blood allele is masked by the A-type blood allele since it is recessive.

I^A i	ii
I^A i	ii

18. D: The building blocks of DNA are nucleotides. A nucleotide is a five-carbon sugar with a phosphate group and a nitrogenous base (Adenine, Guanine, Cytosine, and Thymine). DNA is a double helix and looks like a spiral ladder. Each side has a sugar/phosphate backbone, and the rungs of the ladder that connect the sides are the nitrogen bases. Adenine always pairs with thymine via two hydrogen bonds, and cytosine always pairs with guanine via three hydrogen bonds. The weak hydrogen bonds are important because they allow DNA to easily be opened for replication and transcription.

19. D: There are actually many different types of RNA. The three involved in protein synthesis are messenger RNA (mRNA), ribosomal RNA (rRNA), and transfer RNA (tRNA). Others, including small interfering RNA, micro RNA, and piwi associated RNA, are being investigated. Their known functions include gene regulation, facilitating chromosome wrapping, and unwrapping. RNA, unlike DNA, can be single stranded (mRNA, specifically), has a ribose sugar (rather than deoxyribose, like in DNA), and contains uracil (in place of thymine in DNA).

20. D: Equal sharing of electrons is correct. In water, the electronegative oxygen sucks in the electrons of the two hydrogen atoms, making the oxygen slightly negatively-charged and the hydrogen atoms slightly positively-charged. This unequal sharing is called "polarity." This polarity is responsible for the slightly-positive hydrogen atoms from one molecule being attracted to a slightly-negative oxygen in a different molecule, creating a weak intermolecular force called a hydrogen bond, so *A* and *B* are true. *C* is also true, because this unique hydrogen bonding creates intermolecular forces that literally hold molecules with low enough kinetic energy (at low temperatures) to be held apart at "arm's length" (really, the length of the hydrogen bonds). This makes ice less dense than liquid, which explains why ice floats, a very unique property of water. D is the only statement that is false, so it is the correct answer.

21. D: Cellular respiration is the term used for the set of metabolic reactions that convert chemical bonds to energy in the form of ATP. All respiration starts with glycolysis in the cytoplasm, and in the presence of oxygen, the process will continue to the mitochondria. In a series of oxidation/reduction reactions, primarily glucose will be broken down so that the energy contained within its bonds can be transferred to the smaller ATP molecules. It's like having a $100 bill (glucose) as opposed to having one hundred $1 bills. This is beneficial to the organism because it allows energy to be distributed throughout the cell very easily in smaller packets of energy.

When glucose is broken down, its electrons and hydrogen atoms are involved in oxidative phosphorylation in order to make ATP, while its carbon and oxygen atoms are released as carbon dioxide. Anaerobic respiration does not occur frequently in humans, but during rigorous exercise, lack of available oxygen in the muscles can lead to anaerobic ATP production in a process called lactic acid fermentation. Alcohol fermentation is another type of anaerobic respiration that occurs in yeast. Anaerobic respiration is extremely less efficient than aerobic respiration, as it has a net yield of 2ATP, while aerobic respiration's net yield exceeds 30 ATP.

22. D: All statements are true, but nothing can happen without the message being available; thus, Choice *D* must occur first. After the copy is made in transcription (D), Choice *B* occurs because mRNA has to be processed before being exported into the cytoplasm. Once it has reached the cytoplasm, Choice *A* occurs as mRNA is pulled into the ribosome. Finally, Choice *C* occurs, and tRNA delivers amino acids one at a time until the full polypeptide has been created. At that point, the baby protein (polypeptide) will be processed and folded in the ER and Golgi.

23. B: Punctuated equilibrium is the concept that evolution is comprised of eras of no change, (called "stasis") peppered with short period of rapid change, often resulting in speciation. The theory was researched and proposed by Stephen J. Gould and Niles Eldridge in opposition to Darwin's idea of gradualism. Gradualism maintains that evolution progresses at a steady, gradual pace without sudden new developments.

24. A: All the other answer choices are functions of lipids. *B* is true because steroid hormones are lipid based. Long-term energy is one of the most important functions of lipids, so *C* is true. *D* is also true because the cell membrane is not only composed of a lipid bilayer, but it also has cholesterol (another lipid) embedded within it to regulate membrane fluidity.

25. D: Ribosomes are the structures responsible for protein synthesis using amino acids delivered by tRNA molecules. They are numerous within the cell and can take up as much as 25% of the cell. Ribosomes are found free-floating in the cytoplasm and also attached to the rough endoplasmic reticulum, which resides alongside the nucleus. Ribosomes translate messenger RNA into chains of amino acids that become proteins. Ribosomes themselves are made of protein as well as rRNA. Choice *B* might be an attractive choice, since the Golgi is the site of protein maturation; however, it is not where proteins are synthesized. Choice *A* might be an attractive choice as well because DNA provides the instructions for proteins to be made, but DNA does not make the protein itself.

Chemistry

1. D: 0.01. Scientific notation is always in base 10, and it is a convention used by scientists to express extremely small or large numbers. The first number, referred to as the coefficient, is always greater than or equal to 1 and less than 10. The notation is to multiply the coefficient by a factor of the base, 10. For numbers less than 1, 10 is factored by negative exponent:

$(.02 = 2 \times 10^{-2})$. For numbers greater than 1, the exponent would be positive: $(2,000 = 2 \times 10^{3})$.

2. A: The metric prefix for 10^{-3} is "milli." 10^{-3} is $1/10^3$ or $1/1000$ or 0.001. If this were grams, 10^{-3} would represent 1 milligram or $1/1000$ of a gram. For multiples of 10, the prefixes are as follows: deca = 10^1, hecta = 10^2, kilo = 10^3, mega = 10^6, giga = 10^9, tera = 10^{12}, peta = 10^{15}, and so on. For sub-units of 10, the prefixes are as follows: deci=10^{-1}, centi=10^{-2}, milli=10^{-3}, micro=1^{-6}, nano=10^{-9}, pico=10^{-12}, femto=10^{-15}, and so on. Metric units are usually abbreviated by using the first letter of the prefix (except for micro, which is the Greek letter mu, or μ). Abbreviations for multiples greater than 10^3 are capitalized.

3. B: The conversion from Celsius to Fahrenheit is $°F = \frac{9}{5}(°C) + 32$. Substituting the value for °C gives $°F = \frac{9}{5}(35) + 32$ which yields 95°F. The other choices do not apply the formula correctly and completely.

4. B: Choices A and D both suggest a different number of protons, which would make a different element. It would no longer be a sodium atom if the proton number or atomic number were different, so those are both incorrect. An atom that has a different number of electrons is called an ion, so choice C is incorrect as well.

5. B: They form covalent bonds. If nonmetals form ionic bonds, they will fill their electron orbital (and become an anion) rather than lose electrons (and become a cation), due to their smaller atomic radius and higher electronegativity than metals. A is, therefore, incorrect. There are some nonmetals that are diatomic (hydrogen, oxygen, nitrogen, and halogens), but that is not true for all of them; thus, D is incorrect. Organic compounds are carbon-based due to carbon's ability to form four covalent bonds. In addition to carbon, organic compounds are also rich in hydrogen, phosphorous, nitrogen, oxygen, and sulfur, so C is incorrect as well.

6. B: The basic unit of matter is the atom. Each element is identified by a letter symbol for that element and an atomic number, which indicates the number of protons in that element. Atoms are the building block of each element and are comprised of a nucleus that contains protons (positive charge) and neutrons (no charge). Orbiting around the nucleus at varying distances are negatively-charged electrons. An electrically-neutral atom contains equal numbers of protons and electrons. Atomic mass is the combined mass of protons and neutrons in the nucleus. Electrons have such negligible mass that they are not considered in the atomic mass. Although the nucleus is compact, the electrons orbit in energy levels at great relative distances to it, making an atom mostly empty space.

7. A: Nuclear reactions involve the nucleus, and chemical reactions involve electron behavior alone. If electrons are transferred between atoms, they form ionic bonds. If they are shared between atoms, they form covalent bonds. Unequal sharing within a covalent bond results in intermolecular attractions, including hydrogen bonding. Metallic bonding involves a "sea of electrons," where they float around non-specifically, resulting in metal ductility and malleability, due to their glue-like effect of sticking neighboring atoms together. Their metallic bonding also contributes to electrical conductivity and low specific heats, due to electrons' quick response to charge and heat, given to their mobility. Their floating also results in metals' property of luster as light reflects off the mobile electrons. Electron movement in any type of bond is enhanced by photon and heat energy investments, increasing their likelihood to jump energy levels. Valence electron status is the ultimate contributor to electron behavior as it determines their likelihood to be transferred or shared.

8. A: Electrons give atoms their negative charge. Electron behavior determines their bonding, and bonding can either be covalent (electrons are shared) or ionic (electrons are transferred). The charge of an atom is determined by the electrons in its orbitals. Electrons give atoms their chemical and electromagnetic properties. Unequal numbers of protons and electrons lend either a positive or negative charge to the atom. Ions are atoms with a charge, either positive or negative.

9. B: On the periodic table, the elements are grouped in columns according to the configuration of electrons in their outer orbitals. The groupings on the periodic table give a broad view of trends in chemical properties for the elements. The outer electron shell (or orbital) is most important in determining the chemical properties of the element. The electrons in this orbital determine charge and bonding compatibility. The number of electron shells increases by row from top to bottom. The periodic table is organized with elements that have similar chemical behavior in the columns (groups or families).

10. B: In chemical equations, the reactants are on the left side of the arrow. The direction of the reaction is in the direction of the arrow, although sometimes reactions will be shown with arrows in both directions, meaning the reaction is reversible. The reactants are on the left, and the products of the reaction are on the right side of the arrow. Chemical equations indicate atomic and molecular bond formations, rearrangements, and dissolutions. The numbers in front of the elements are called coefficients, and they designate the number of moles of that element accounted for in the reaction. The subscript numbers tell how many atoms of that element are in the molecule, with the number "1" being understood. In H_2O, for example, there are two atoms of hydrogen bound to one atom of oxygen. The ionic charge of the element is shown in superscripts and can be either positive or negative.

11. B: The law of conservation of mass states that matter can not be created or destroyed, but that it can change forms. This is important in balancing chemical equations on both sides of the arrow. Unbalanced equations will have an unequal number of atoms of each element on either side of the equation and violate the law.

12. D: Solids all increase solubility with choices A-C. Powdered hot chocolate is an example to consider. Heating (*A*) and stirring (*B*) make it dissolve faster. Regarding Choice *C*, powder is in chunks that collectively result in a very large surface area, as opposed to a chocolate bar that has a very small relative surface area. The small, surface area form dramatically increases solubility. Decreasing the solvent (most of the time, water) will decrease solubility.

13. A: The quantity of a solute in a solution can be calculated by multiplying the molarity of the solution by the volume. The equivalence point is the point at which an unknown solute has completely reacted with a known solute concentration. The limiting reactant is the reactant completely consumed by a reaction. The theoretical yield is the quantity of product produced by a reaction.

14. A: When salt is added to water, it increases its boiling point. This is an example of a colligative property, which is any property that changes the physical property of a substance. This particular colligative property of boiling point elevation occurs because the extra solute dissolved in water reduces the surface area of the water, impeding it from vaporizing. If heat is applied, though, it gives water particles enough kinetic energy to vaporize. This additional heat results in an increased boiling point. Other colligative properties of solutions include the following: their melting points decrease with the addition of solute, and their osmotic pressure increases (because it creates a concentration gradient that was otherwise not there).

15. C: Pressure has little effect on the solubility of a liquid solution because liquid is not easily compressible; therefore, increased pressure won't result in increased kinetic energy. Pressure increases solubility in gaseous solutions, since it causes them to move faster.

16. B: Nonpolar molecules have hydrophobic regions that do not dissolve in water. Oil is a nonpolar molecule that repels water. Polar molecules combine readily with water, which is, itself, a polar solvent. Polar molecules are hydrophilic or "water-loving" because their polar regions have intermolecular bonding with water via hydrogen bonds. Some structures and molecules are both polar and nonpolar, like the phospholipid bilayer. The phospholipid bilayer has polar heads that are the external "water-loving portions" and hydrophobic tails that are immiscible in water. Polar solvents dissolve polar solutes, and nonpolar solvents dissolve nonpolar solutes. One way to remember these is "Like dissolves like."

17. A: A catalyst increases the rate of a chemical reaction by lowering the activation energy. Enzymes are biological protein catalysts that are utilized by organisms to facilitate anabolic and catabolic reactions. They speed up the rate of reaction by making the reaction easier (perhaps by orienting a molecule more favorably upon induced fit, for example). Catalysts are not used up by the reaction and can be used over and over again.

18. C: Proteins are made up of chains of amino acids. Lipids are usually nonpolar, hydrophobic molecules. Nucleic acids are made of nucleotides. Carbohydrates are ring-like molecules built using carbon, oxygen, and hydrogen.

19. C: 2: 9:10:4. These are the coefficients that follow the law of conservation of matter. The coefficient times the subscript of each element should be the same on both sides of the equation.

20. A: Ionic bonding is the result of electrons transferred between atoms. When an atom loses one or more electrons, a cation, or positively-charged ion, is formed. An anion, or negatively-charged ion, is formed when an atom gains one or more electrons. Ionic bonds are formed from the attraction between a positively-charged cation and a negatively-charged anion. The bond between sodium and chloride in table salt or sodium chloride, Na^+Cl^-, is an example of an ionic bond.

21. A: Oxidation is when a substance loses electrons in a chemical reaction, and reduction is when a substance gains electrons. Any element by itself has a charge of 0, as iron and oxygen do on the reactant side. In the ionic compound formed, iron has a +3 charge, and oxygen has a -2 charge. Because iron had a zero charge that then changed to +3, it means that it lost three electrons and was oxidized. Oxygen that gained two electrons was reduced.

22. C: Fission occurs when heavy nuclei are split and is currently the energy source that fuels power plants. Fusion, on the other hand, is the combining of small nuclei and produces far more energy, and it is the nuclear reaction that powers stars like the sun. Harnessing the extreme energy released by fusion has proven impossible so far, which is unfortunate since its waste products are not radioactive, while waste produced by fission typically is.

23. A: Alpha decay involves a helium particle emission (with two neutrons). Beta decay involves emission of an electron or positron, and gamma is just high-energy light emissions.

24. B: Choice *A* is false because it is possible to have a very strong acid with a pH between 0 and 1. *C* is false because the pH scale is from 0 to 14, and -2 is outside the boundaries. *D* is false because a solution with a pH of 2 has ten times fewer hydronium ions than a pH of 1 solution.

25. C: Gamma is the lightest radioactive decay with the most energy, and this high energy is toxic to cells. Due to its weightlessness, gamma rays are extremely penetrating. Alpha particles are heavy and can be easily shielded by skin. Beta particles are electrons and can penetrate more than an alpha particle because they are lighter. Beta particles can be shielded by plastic.

Anatomy and Physiology

1. A: When activated, B cells create antibodies against specific antigens. White blood cells are generated in yellow bone marrow, not cartilage. Platelets are not a type of white blood cell and are typically cell fragments produced by megakaryocytes. White blood cells are active throughout nearly all of one's life and have not been shown to specially activate or deactivate because of life events like puberty or menopause.

2. D: Mechanical digestion is physical digestion of food and tearing it into smaller pieces using force. This occurs in the stomach and mouth. Chemical digestion involves chemically changing the food and breaking it down into small organic compounds that can be utilized by the cell to build molecules. The salivary glands in the mouth secrete amylase that breaks down starch, which begins chemical digestion. The stomach contains enzymes such as pepsinogen/pepsin and gastric lipase, which chemically digest protein and fats, respectively. The small intestine continues to digest protein using the enzymes trypsin and chymotrypsin. It also digests fats with the help of bile from the liver and lipase from the pancreas. These organs act as exocrine glands because they secrete substances through a duct. Carbohydrates are digested in the small intestine with the help of pancreatic amylase, gut bacterial flora and fauna, and brush border enzymes like lactose. Brush border enzymes are contained in the towel-like microvilli in the small intestine that soak up nutrients.

3. D: The urinary system has many functions, the primary of which is removing waste products and balancing water and electrolyte concentrations in the blood. It also plays a key role in regulating ion concentrations, such as sodium, potassium, chloride, and calcium, in the filtrate. The urinary system helps maintain blood pH by reabsorbing or secreting hydrogen ions and bicarbonate as necessary. Certain kidney cells can detect reductions in blood volume and pressure and then can secrete renin to activate a hormone that causes increased reabsorption of sodium ions and water. This serves to raise blood volume and pressure. Kidney cells secrete erythropoietin under hypoxic conditions to stimulate red blood cell production. They also synthesize calcitriol, a hormone derivative of vitamin D3, which aids in calcium ion absorption by the intestinal epithelium.

4. C: The blood leaves the right ventricle through a semi-lunar valve and goes through the pulmonary artery to the lungs. Any increase in pressure in the artery will eventually affect the contractibility of the right ventricle. Blood enters the right atrium from the superior and inferior venae cava veins, and blood leaves the right atrium through the tricuspid valve to the right ventricle. Blood enters the left atrium from the pulmonary veins carrying oxygenated blood from the lungs. Blood flows from the left atrium to the left ventricle through the mitral valve and leaves the left ventricle through a semi-lunar valve to enter the aorta.

5. D: Sodium bicarbonate, a very effective base, has the chief function to increase the pH of the chyme. Chyme leaving the stomach has a very low pH, due to the high amounts of acid that are used to digest and break down food. If this is not neutralized, the walls of the small intestine will be damaged and may form ulcers. Sodium bicarb is produced by the pancreas and released in response to pyloric stimulation so that it can neutralize the acid. It has little to no digestive effect.

6. D: A reflex arc is a simple nerve pathway involving a stimulus, a synapse, and a response that is controlled by the spinal cord—not the brain. The knee-jerk reflex is an example of a reflex arc. The stimulus is the hammer touching the tendon, reaching the synapse in the spinal cord by an afferent pathway. The response is the resulting muscle contraction reaching the muscle by an efferent pathway. None of the remaining processes is a simple reflex. Memories are processed and stored in the hippocampus in the limbic system. The visual center is located in the occipital lobe, while auditory processing occurs in the temporal lobe. The sympathetic and parasympathetic divisions of the autonomic nervous system control heart and blood pressure.

7. B: Ligaments connect bone to bone. Tendons connect muscle to bone. Both are made of dense, fibrous connective tissue (primary Type 1 collagen) to give strength. However, tendons are more organized, especially in the long axis direction like muscle fibers themselves, and they have more collagen. This arrangement makes more sense because muscles have specific orientations of their fibers, so they contract in somewhat predictable directions. Ligaments are less organized and more of a woven pattern because bone connections are not as organized as bundles or muscle fibers, so ligaments must have strength in multiple directions to protect against injury.

8. A: The three primary body planes are coronal, sagittal, and transverse. The coronal or frontal plane, named for the plane in which a corona or halo might appear in old paintings, divides the body vertically into front and back sections. The sagittal plane, named for the path an arrow might take when shot at the body, divides the body vertically into right and left sections. The transverse plane divides the body horizontally into upper or superior and lower or inferior sections. There is no medial plane, per se. The anatomical direction medial simply references a location close or closer to the center of the body than another location.

9. C: Although the lungs may provide some cushioning for the heart when the body is violently struck, this is not a major function of the respiratory system. Its most notable function is that of gas exchange for oxygen and carbon dioxide, but it also plays a vital role in the regulation of blood pH. The aqueous form of carbon dioxide, carbonic acid, is a major pH buffer of the blood, and the respiratory system directly controls how much carbon dioxide stays and is released from the blood through respiration. The respiratory system also enables vocalization and forms the basis for the mode of speech and language used by most humans.

10. A: The forebrain contains the cerebrum, the thalamus, the hypothalamus, and the limbic system. The limbic system is chiefly responsible for the perception of emotions through the amygdale, while the cerebrum interprets sensory input and generates movement. Specifically, the occipital lobe receives visual input, and the primary motor cortex in the frontal lobe is the controller of voluntary movement. The hindbrain, specifically the medulla oblongata and brain stem, control and regulate blood pressure and heart rate.

11. C: Nephrons are responsible for filtering blood. When functioning properly they allow blood cells and nutrients to go back into the bloodstream while sending waste to the bladder. However, nephrons can fail at doing this, particularly when blood flood to the kidneys is limited. The medulla (also called the renal medulla) (*A*) and the renal cortex (*D*) are both parts of the kidney but are not specifically responsible for filtering blood. The medulla is in the inner part of the kidney and contains the nephrons. The renal cortex is the outer part of the kidney. The heart (*B*) is responsible for pumping blood throughout the body rather than filtering it.

12. B: Ossification is the process by which cartilage, a soft, flexible substance is replaced by bone throughout the body. All humans regardless of age have cartilage, but cartilage in some areas goes away to make way for bones.

13. D: The seminiferous tubules are responsible for sperm production. Had *testicles* been an answer choice, it would also have been correct since it houses the seminiferous tubules. The prostate gland (*A*) secretes enzymes that help nourish sperm after creation. The seminal vesicles (*B*) secrete some of the components of semen. The scrotum (*C*) is the pouch holding the testicles.

14. C: The parasympathetic nervous system is related to calm, peaceful times without stress that require no immediate decisions. It relaxes the fight-or-flight response, slows heart rate to a comfortable pace, and decreases bronchiole dilation to a normal size. The sympathetic nervous system, on the other hand, is in charge of the fight-or-flight response and works to increase blood pressure and oxygen absorption.

15. C: The parathryroid gland impacts calcium levels by secreting parathyroid hormone (PTH). Osteotoid gland is not a real gland. The pineal gland regulates sleep by secreting melatonin, and the thymus gland focuses on immunity. *Thyroid* would also be a correct answer choice as it influences the levels of circulating calcium.

16. B: For measuring blood, we're looking for a unit that measure volume. Choice *A*, *B*, and *C* are all measures of volume, but pounds (*D*) is a measure of weight. The correct answer is liters, as the average adult has about 5 liters of blood in their body. Blood can certainly be measured in ounces or milliliters; however, 5 liters is equal to 5,000 milliliters or 176 ounces. Thus, liters seems to be the more rational measuring unit.

17. D: Arteries carry oxygen-rich blood from the heart to the other tissues of the body. Veins carry oxygen-poor blood back to the heart. Intestines carry digested food through the body. Bronchioles are passageways that carry air from the nose and mouth to the lungs.

18. C: The somatic nervous system is the voluntary nervous system, responsible for voluntary movement. It includes nerves that transmit signals from the brain to the muscles of the body. Breathing is controlled by the autonomic nervous system. Thought and fear are complex processes that occur in the brain, which is part of the central nervous system.

19. A: Platelets are the blood components responsible for clotting. There are between 150,000 and 450,000 platelets in healthy blood. When a clot forms, platelets adhere to the injured area of the vessel and promote a molecular cascade that results in adherence of more platelets. Ultimately, the platelet aggregation results in recruitment of a protein called fibrin, which adds structure to the clot. Too many platelets can cause clotting disorders. Not enough leads to bleeding disorders.

20. C: The sinuses function to warm, filter, and humidify air that is inhaled. Choice *A* is incorrect because mucus traps airborne pathogens. Choice *B* is incorrect because the epiglottis is the structure in the pharynx that covers the trachea during swallowing to prevent food from entering it. Lastly, Choice *D*, sweeping away pathogens and directing them toward the top of the trachea, is the function of cilia. Respiratory structures, such as the nasal passages and trachea, are lined with mucus and cilia.

21. A: The renal pelvis acts like funnel by delivering the urine from the millions of the collecting tubules to the ureters. It is the most central part of the kidney. The renal cortex is the outer layer of the kidney, while the renal medulla is the inner layer. The renal medulla contains the functional units of the kidneys—nephrons—which function to filter the blood. Choice *D*, Bowman's capsule, is the name for the structure that covers the glomeruli.

22. C: A cluster of capillaries that functions as the main filter of the blood entering the kidney is known as the glomerulus, so Choice *C* is correct. The Bowman's capsule surrounds the glomerulus and receives fluid and solutes from it; therefore, Choice *A* is incorrect. The loop of Henle is a part of the kidney tubule where water and nutrients are reabsorbed, so *B* is false. The nephron is the unit containing all of these anatomical features, making Choice *D* incorrect as well.

23. C: The alveoli are small sac-shaped structures at the end of the bronchioles where gas exchange takes place. The bronchioles are tubes through which air travels. The kidneys and medulla oblongata do not directly affect oxygen and carbon dioxide exchange.

24. C: The uterus and ovaries aren't part of the birth canal, so Choices *A* and *D* are false. The cervix is the uppermost portion of the birth canal, so Choice *B* is incorrect, making Choice *C* the correct answer, as the vagina is the muscular tube on the lowermost portion of the birth canal that connects the exterior environment to the cervix.

25. C: The pancreas functions as an exocrine gland because it secretes enzymes that break down food components. It also functions as an endocrine gland because it secretes hormones that regulate blood sugar levels. The kidney isn't a gland; it is an organ located directly below the adrenal glands. The stomach is an exocrine gland because it secretes hydrochloric acid. Like the kidney, the spleen is an organ, not a gland. Therefore, the only correct answer is *C*.

Physics

1. A: Velocity is a measure of speed with direction. To calculate velocity, find the distance covered and the time it took to cover that distance; change in position over the change in time. A standard measurement for velocity is in meters per second (m/s). The change in speed over change in time is acceleration, while acceleration with direction has no specific name.

2. B: Acceleration is the rate of change in velocity. Speed is the rate at which an object moves, velocity is speed in a given direction, and momentum is the velocity of an object multiplied by its mass.

3. B: While this is an important brainchild of Einstein's general relativity, it is not one of Newton's original three laws of motion. Newton's three laws are describe how a force is defined as how much a mass is accelerated, how an object resists changes in inertia, and how all forces act with an equal and opposite reaction.

4. C: This is the actual force recognized in a rotational situation. The reactive force acting opposite of the centripetal force is named the centrifugal force, but it is not an actual force on its own. A common mistake is to interchange the two terms. The real force acting in a rotational situation is pulling in toward the axis of rotation and is called the centripetal force. Gravity technically only acts between all mass, so it is not specific enough for the question.

5. B: Kinetic energy is energy an object has while moving; potential energy is energy an object has based on its position or height. Electric and electromagnetic energies are other descriptions of generally potential energy contained in waves or fields, but neither has anything directly to do with movement.

6. B: Waves are periodic disturbances in a gas, liquid, or solid as energy is transmitted. Waves don't carry or slow down matter, but instead transfer energy.

7. A: The definition of refraction is when a wave bends (such as when the medium it is traveling through changes). Diffraction is when a wave bends around an object (such as when the medium it is traveling through runs into a barrier), so is too specific an answer for the question. Reflection is when a wave bounces off a surface without losing energy or becoming distorted, and convection is the thermal energy transferred through gases and liquids by convection currents.

8. A: Protons and neutrons are both found in the atomic nucleus, while electrons move freely in the electron cloud of an atom. Ions are a different name for entire atoms with unequal numbers of protons and electrons; since this includes electrons, it cannot describe things solely found in the nucleus (unless you were visualizing a hydrogen ion, which is a particular case and is arguably not general enough for the question).

9. C: Electricity moves from objects with greater potential energy to objects with less potential energy. Similarly to how warm air spreads towards colder environments or how gasses and liquids move from areas of high concentration to areas of low concentration, electric currents are generated by the electric field moving electrons from areas of high voltage potential to areas of low voltage potential.

10. A: The recurring theme in electricity and magnetism is that like, similar, or identical charges repel one another (whether it is two negative charges or two positive charges) while unlike, dissimilar, or different charges attract one another. This is exemplified by Coulomb's law, which states that charges of the same sign produce a positive force (which repels the particles) and that charges of opposite signs produce a negative force (which attracts the particles).

Dear HESI Admission Assessment Test Taker,

We would like to start by thanking you for purchasing this study guide for your HESI exam. We hope that we exceeded your expectations.

Our goal in creating this study guide was to cover all of the topics that you will see on the test. We also strove to make our practice questions as similar as possible to what you will encounter on test day. With that being said, if you found something that you feel was not up to your standards, please send us an email and let us know.

We would also like to let you know about other books in our catalog that may interest you.

ATI TEAS 6

This can be found on Amazon: amazon.com/dp/162845427X

CEN

amazon.com/dp/1628454768

We have study guides in a wide variety of fields. If the one you are looking for isn't listed above, then try searching for it on Amazon or send us an email.

Thanks Again and Happy Testing!
Product Development Team
info@studyguideteam.com

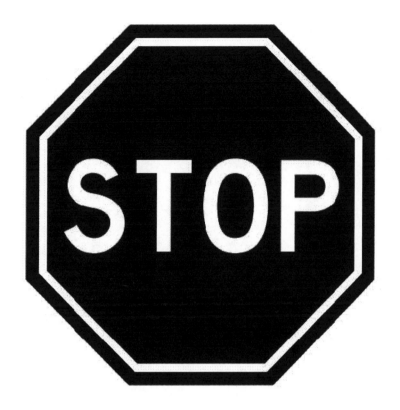

FREE Test Taking Tips DVD Offer

To help us better serve you, we have developed a Test Taking Tips DVD that we would like to give you for FREE. **This DVD covers world-class test taking tips that you can use to be even more successful when you are taking your test.**

All that we ask is that you email us your feedback about your study guide. Please let us know what you thought about it – whether that is good, bad or indifferent.

To get your **FREE Test Taking Tips DVD**, email freedvd@studyguideteam.com with "FREE DVD" in the subject line and the following information in the body of the email:

    a. The title of your study guide.

    b. Your product rating on a scale of 1-5, with 5 being the highest rating.

    c. Your feedback about the study guide. What did you think of it?

    d. Your full name and shipping address to send your free DVD.

If you have any questions or concerns, please don't hesitate to contact us at freedvd@studyguideteam.com.